Healthy and Delicious:

25 Diet Recipes for Every Meal

Table of Contents

Introduction

The Importance of a Balanced Diet

A balanced diet is essential for maintaining a healthy weight, boosting energy, and preventing chronic diseases. This book offers 30 diet recipes that focus on wholesome ingredients, portion control, and flavor, ensuring that you enjoy your meals while nourishing your body.

Tips for Healthy Cooking

1. **Use Whole Ingredients:** Opt for whole grains, lean proteins, fresh vegetables, and healthy fats.
2. **Minimize Processed Foods:** Avoid processed sugars, refined flours, and unhealthy fats.

3. **Control Portions:** Understanding serving sizes helps prevent overeating.

4. **Flavor with Herbs and Spices:** Enhance taste without extra calories by using fresh herbs and spices.

5. **Cook at Home:** Home-cooked meals are often healthier than takeout or restaurant dishes.

Understanding Portions and Calorie Counts

Balancing calories consumed with calories burned is key to weight management. Each recipe in this book includes calorie information to help you stay on track.

Breakfast Recipes

Recipe 1: Avocado Toast with Poached Egg

Ingredients:

- 1 slice whole grain bread
- ½ ripe avocado
- 1 large egg
- 1 tsp lemon juice
- Salt and pepper to taste
- Optional: Red pepper flakes, fresh herbs

Instructions:

1. **Toast the Bread:** Toast the whole grain bread until it's crispy and golden brown.

2. **Prepare the Avocado:** Mash the avocado in a small bowl with lemon juice, salt, and pepper.
3. **Poach the Egg:** Bring a pot of water to a gentle simmer. Crack the egg into a small bowl, then gently slide it into the water. Cook for 3-4 minutes until the whites are set and the yolk is still runny.
4. **Assemble the Toast:** Spread the mashed avocado on the toast, top with the poached egg, and sprinkle with red pepper flakes or fresh herbs if desired.

Nutritional Information (per serving):

- Calories: 250
- Protein: 10g
- Fat: 18g
- Carbohydrates: 20g
- Fiber: 7g

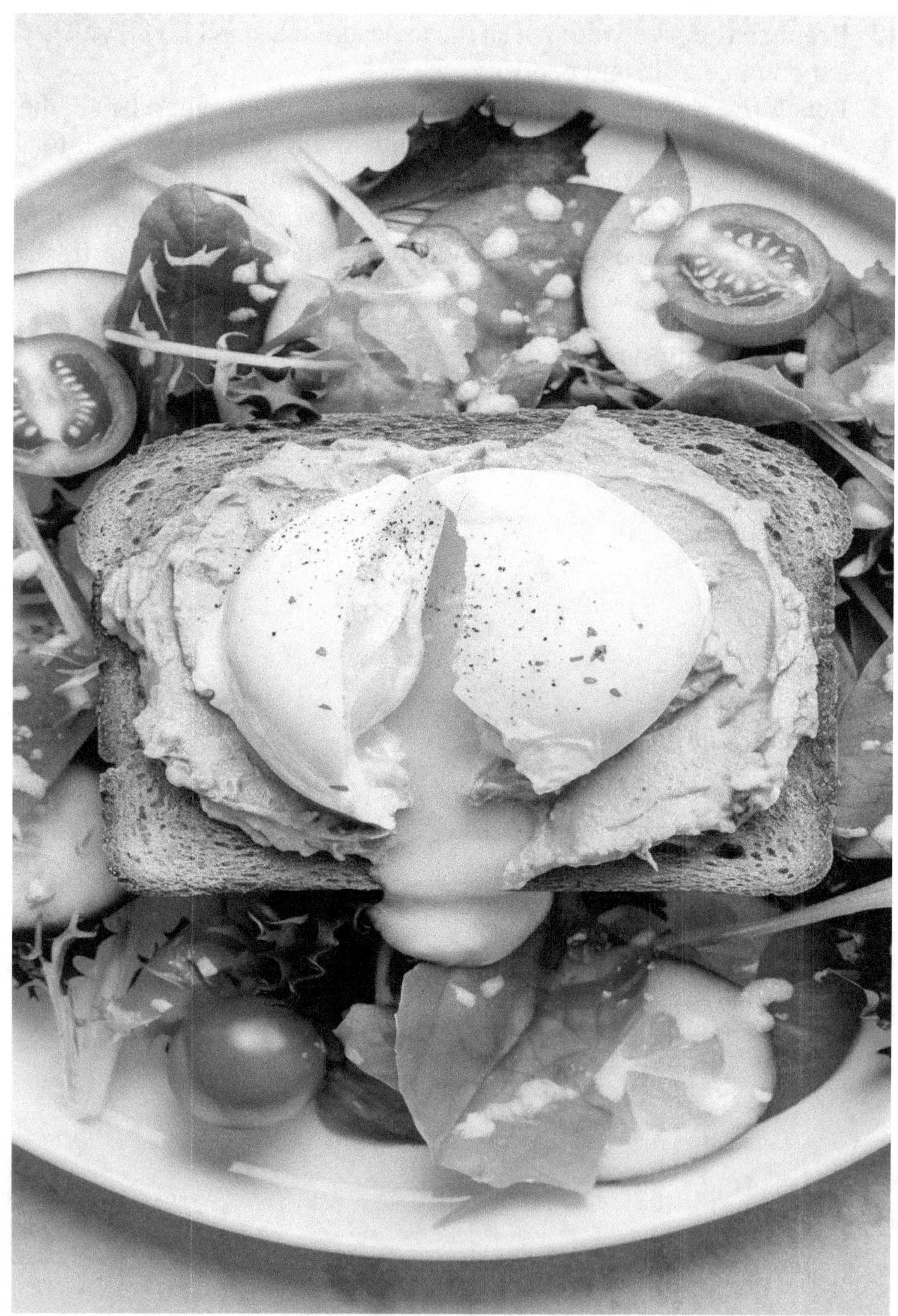

Recipe 2: Greek Yogurt Parfait with Berries

Ingredients:

- 1 cup Greek yogurt (plain or vanilla)
- ½ cup mixed berries (strawberries, blueberries, raspberries)
- 1 tbsp honey
- ¼ cup granola
- Optional: Chia seeds, nuts

Instructions:

1. **Layer the Yogurt:** Spoon half of the yogurt into a bowl or glass.
2. **Add the Berries:** Top with a layer of mixed berries.
3. **Drizzle with Honey:** Drizzle half of the honey over the berries.
4. **Add Granola:** Sprinkle granola on top of the berries.
5. **Repeat:** Add another layer of yogurt, berries, honey, and granola.
6. **Optional:** Top with chia seeds or nuts for added texture and nutrition.

Nutritional Information (per serving):

- Calories: 300
- Protein: 15g
- Fat: 8g
- Carbohydrates: 45g
- Fiber: 6g

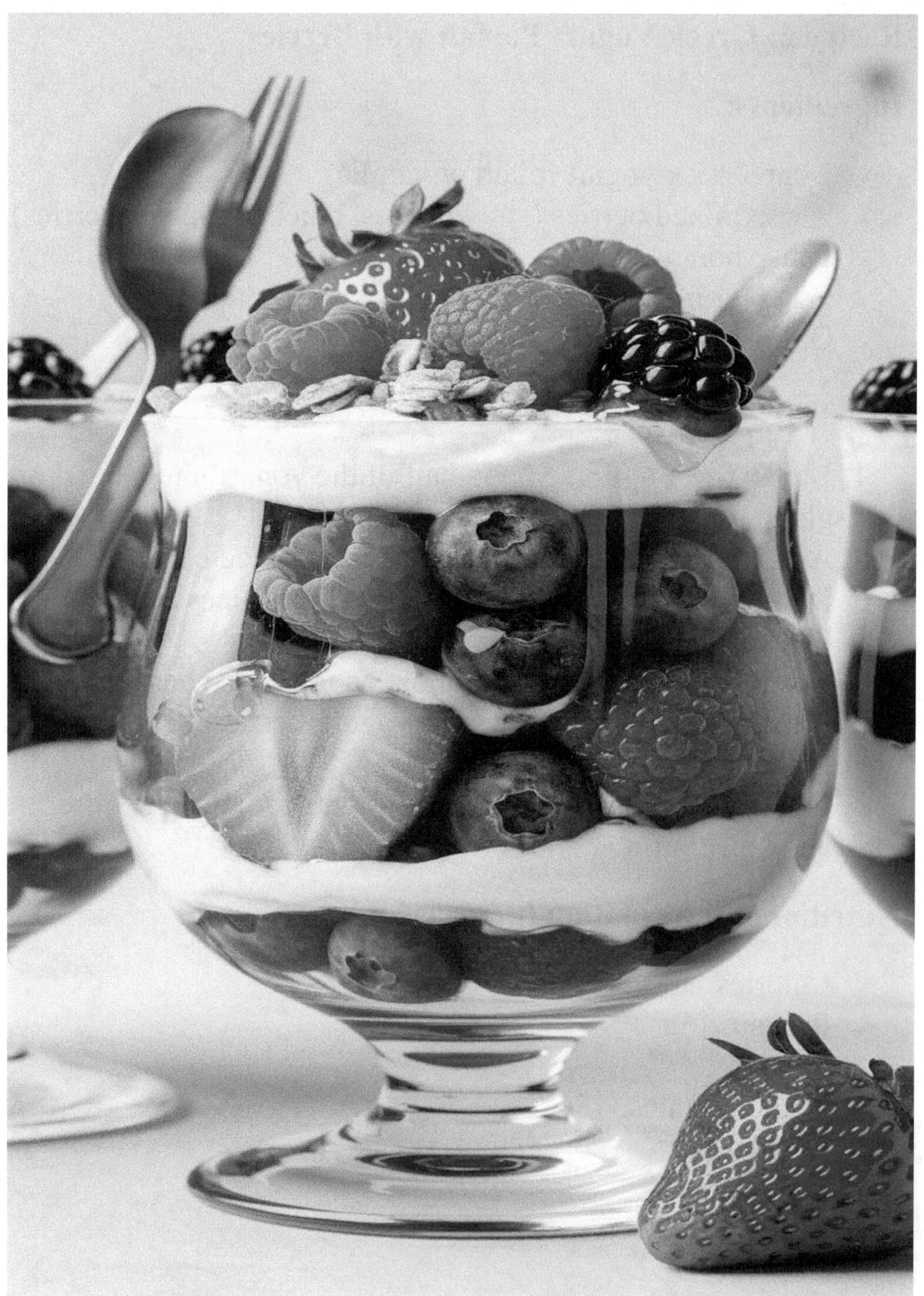

Recipe 3: Spinach and Mushroom Omelet

Ingredients:

- 2 large eggs
- ½ cup spinach, chopped
- ¼ cup mushrooms, sliced
- 1 tbsp olive oil
- Salt and pepper to taste
- Optional: Cheese, herbs

Instructions:

1. **Sauté the Vegetables:** Heat olive oil in a non-stick pan over medium heat. Add the mushrooms and cook until softened. Add the spinach and cook until wilted.
2. **Beat the Eggs:** In a bowl, whisk the eggs with salt and pepper.
3. **Cook the Omelette:** Pour the eggs over the spinach and mushrooms in the pan. Cook until the eggs are set, then fold the omelette in half.
4. **Serve:** Slide the omelette onto a plate and serve immediately.

Nutritional Information (per serving):

- Calories: 200
- Protein: 12g
- Fat: 15g
- Carbohydrates: 4g
- Fiber: 2g

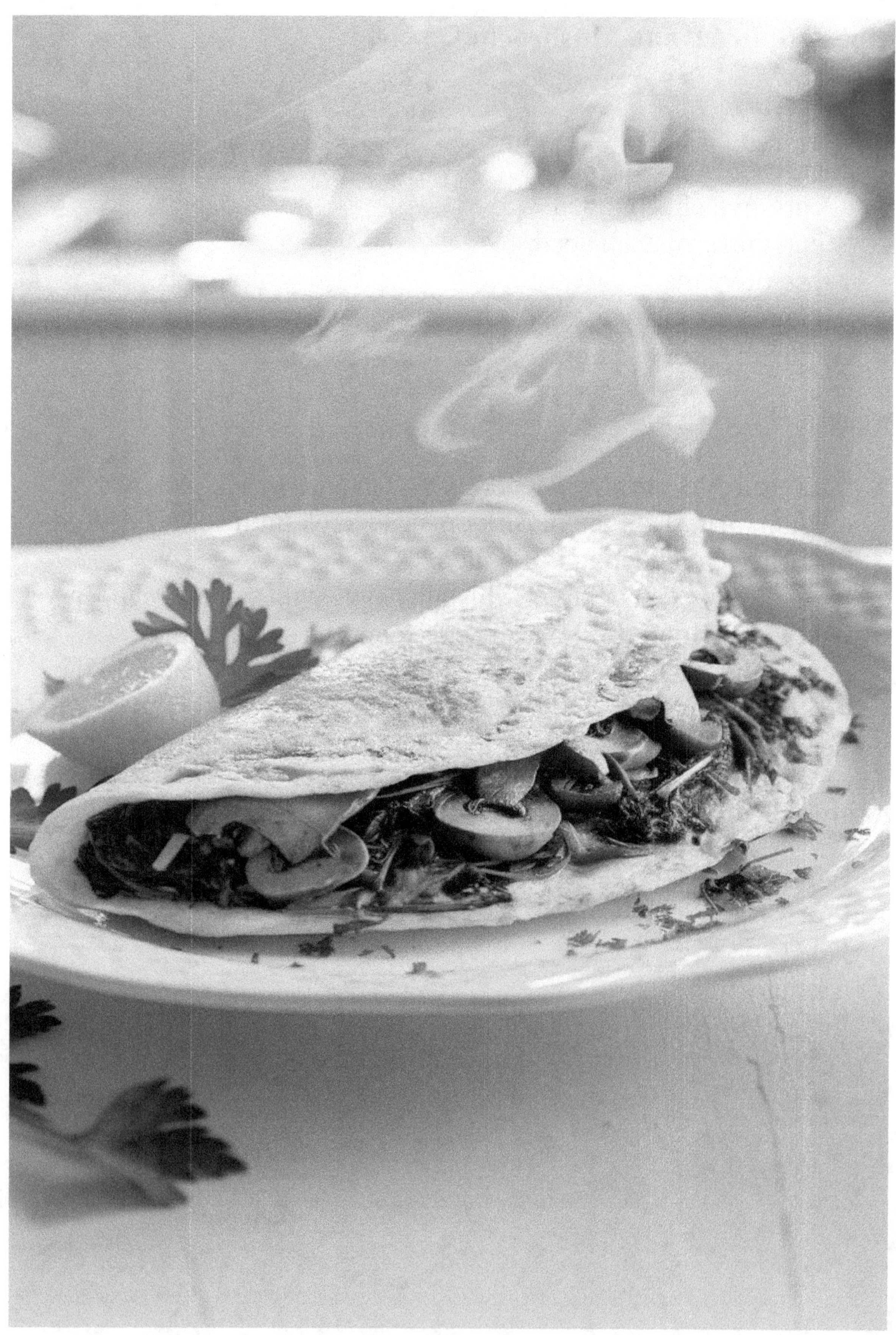

Recipe 4: Overnight Oats with Chia Seeds

Ingredients:

- ½ cup rolled oats
- 1 tbsp chia seeds
- 1 cup almond milk (or any milk of choice)
- 1 tbsp honey or maple syrup
- Fruit toppings (e.g., berries, banana slices, or diced apple)
- Optional: Nuts, seeds, cinnamon

Instructions:

1. **Mix Ingredients:** In a mason jar or bowl, combine oats, chia seeds, milk, and honey. Stir well.
2. **Refrigerate Overnight:** Cover and refrigerate overnight, or for at least 4 hours, to allow the oats and chia seeds to soak and soften.
3. **Add Toppings:** In the morning, top with your favorite fruit, nuts, or seeds. Sprinkle with cinnamon if desired.

Nutritional Information (per serving):

- Calories: 300
- Protein: 8g
- Fat: 10g
- Carbohydrates: 45g
- Fiber: 10g

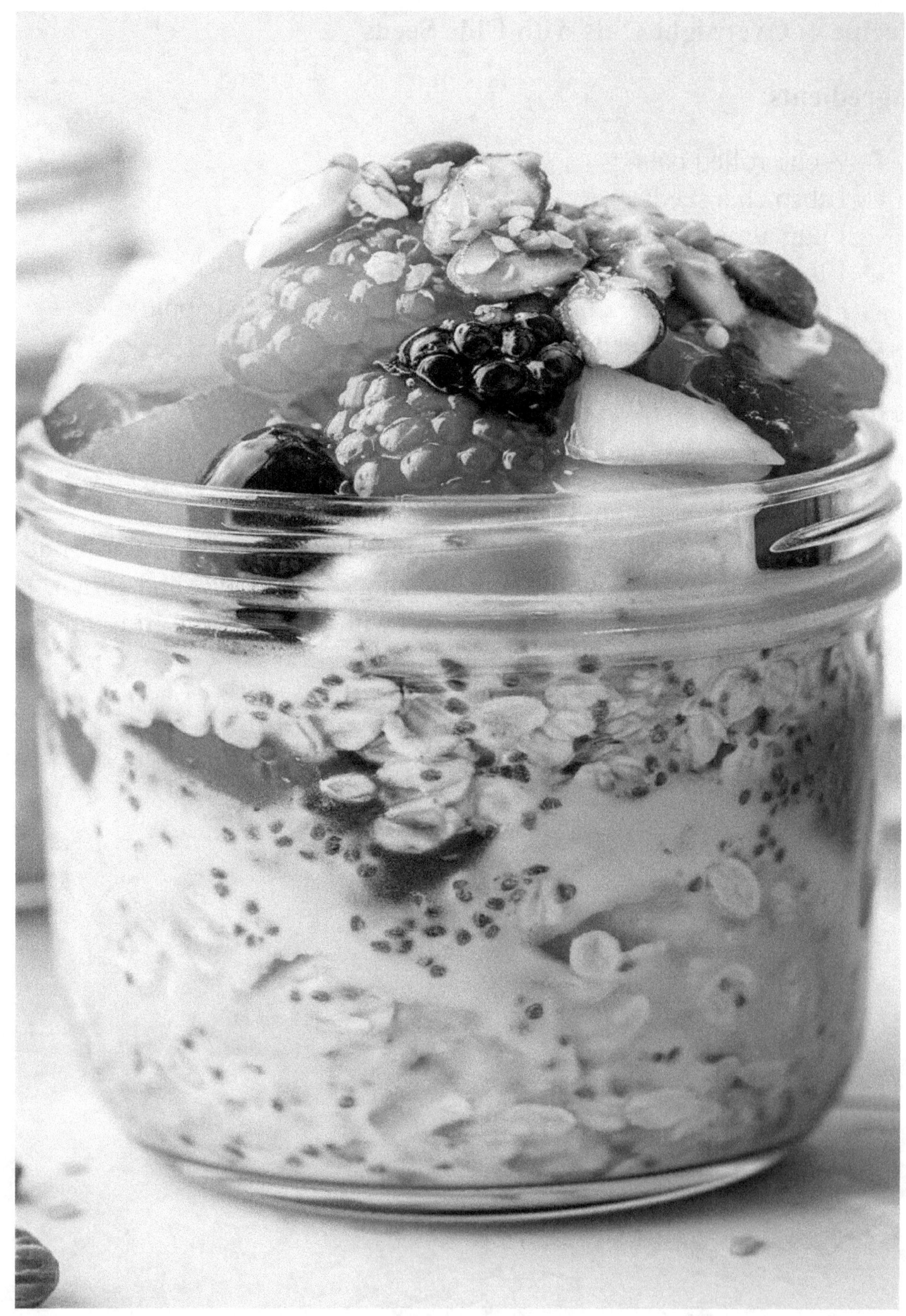

Recipe 5: Smoothie Bowl

Ingredients:

- 1 cup frozen mixed berries
- 1 banana, sliced
- 1 cup spinach
- ½ cup almond milk (or any milk of choice)
- ¼ cup granola
- Toppings: Fresh fruit, nuts, seeds, coconut flakes

Instructions:

1. **Blend the Smoothie:** In a blender, combine the frozen berries, banana, spinach, and milk. Blend until smooth and thick.
2. **Pour into a Bowl:** Pour the smoothie into a bowl.
3. **Add Toppings:** Top with granola, fresh fruit, nuts, seeds, or coconut flakes.

Nutritional Information (per serving):

- Calories: 350
- Protein: 8g
- Fat: 12g
- Carbohydrates: 55g
- Fiber: 12g

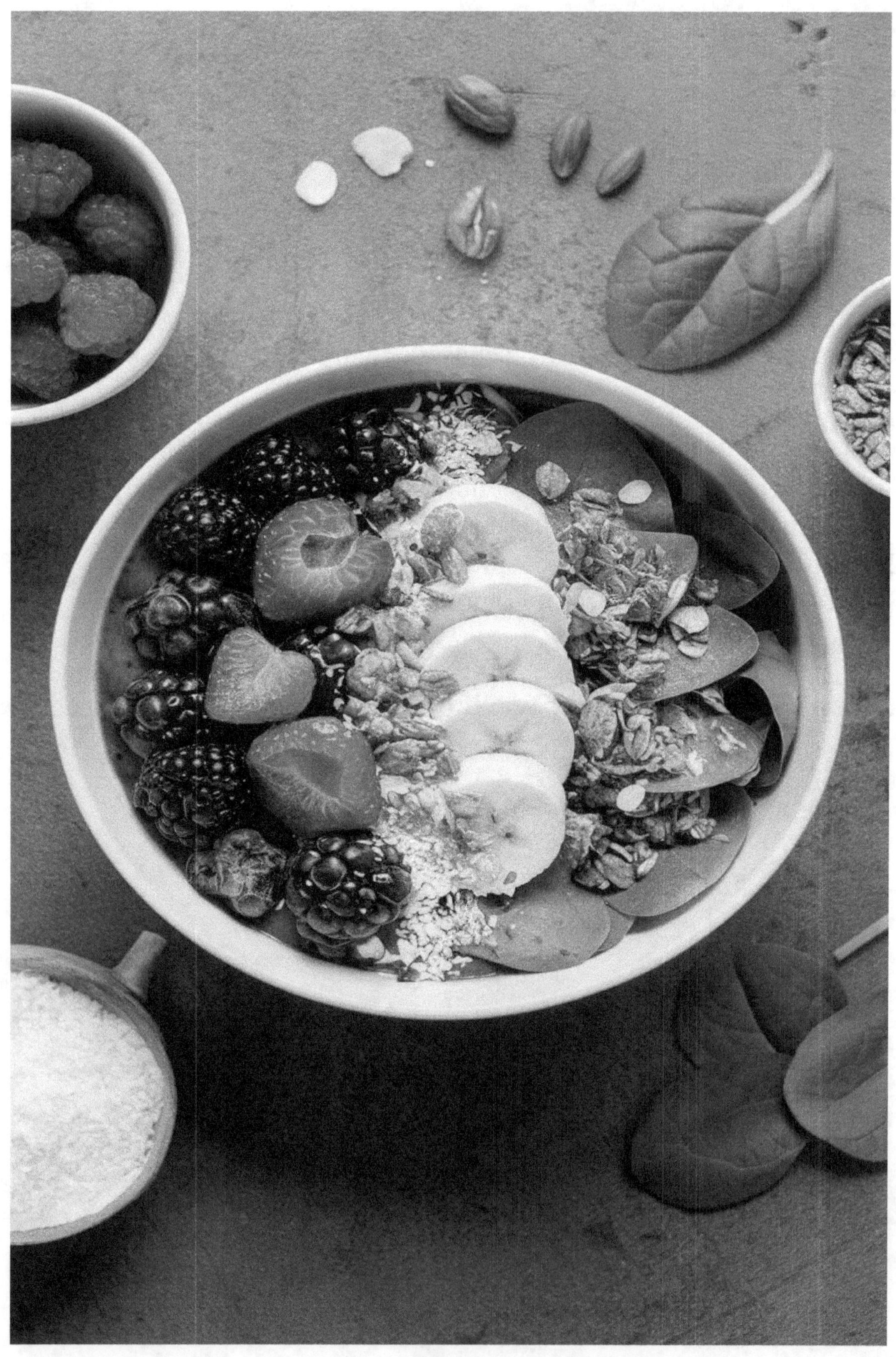

Lunch Recipes

Recipe 6: Quinoa Salad with Grilled Chicken

Ingredients:

- 1 cup quinoa, cooked
- 1 grilled chicken breast, sliced
- 1 cucumber, diced
- 1 cup cherry tomatoes, halved
- ¼ cup feta cheese, crumbled
- 2 tbsp lemon vinaigrette (lemon juice, olive oil, Dijon mustard)
- Optional: Fresh herbs (parsley, mint)

Instructions:

1. **Cook Quinoa:** Rinse quinoa under cold water. Cook according to package instructions. Allow to cool.
2. **Grill the Chicken:** Season chicken with salt and pepper. Grill until fully cooked, then slice.
3. **Prepare the Vegetables:** Dice

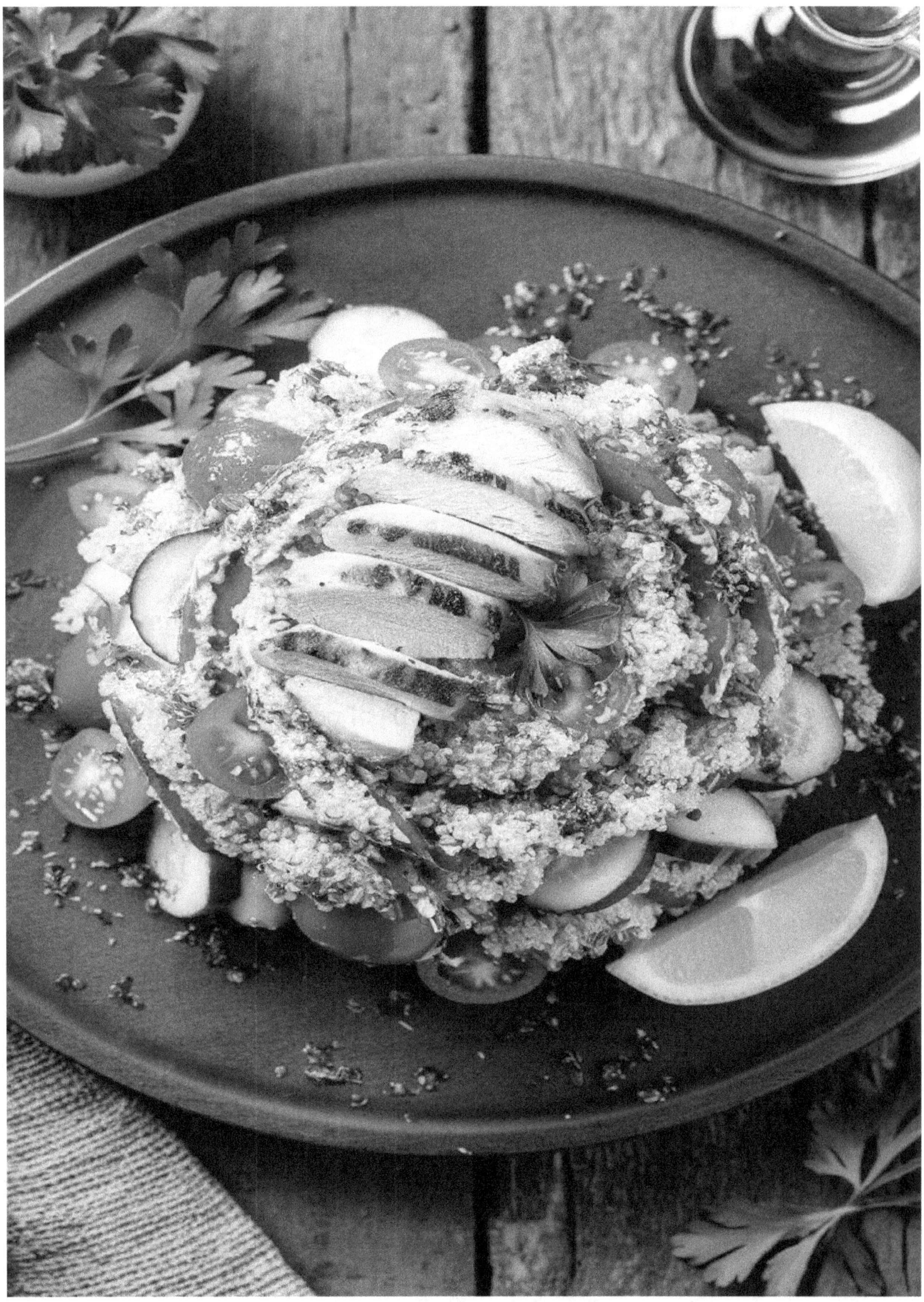

Recipe 7: Zucchini Noodles with Pesto

Ingredients:

- 2 medium zucchinis, spiralized into noodles
- ¼ cup basil pesto
- 1 cup cherry tomatoes, halved
- ¼ cup Parmesan cheese, grated
- 1 tbsp olive oil
- Optional: Pine nuts, fresh basil

Instructions:

1. **Spiralize the Zucchini:** Use a spiralizer to create zucchini noodles. Set aside.
2. **Sauté the Zoodles:** Heat olive oil in a pan over medium heat. Add zucchini noodles and cook for 2-3 minutes until slightly softened.
3. **Add Pesto:** Toss the zoodles with basil pesto until evenly coated.
4. **Add Tomatoes:** Stir in the cherry tomatoes and cook for another minute.
5. **Serve:** Garnish with Parmesan cheese, pine nuts, and fresh basil.

Nutritional Information (per serving):

- Calories: 300
- Protein: 10g
- Fat: 22g
- Carbohydrates: 15g
- Fiber: 5g

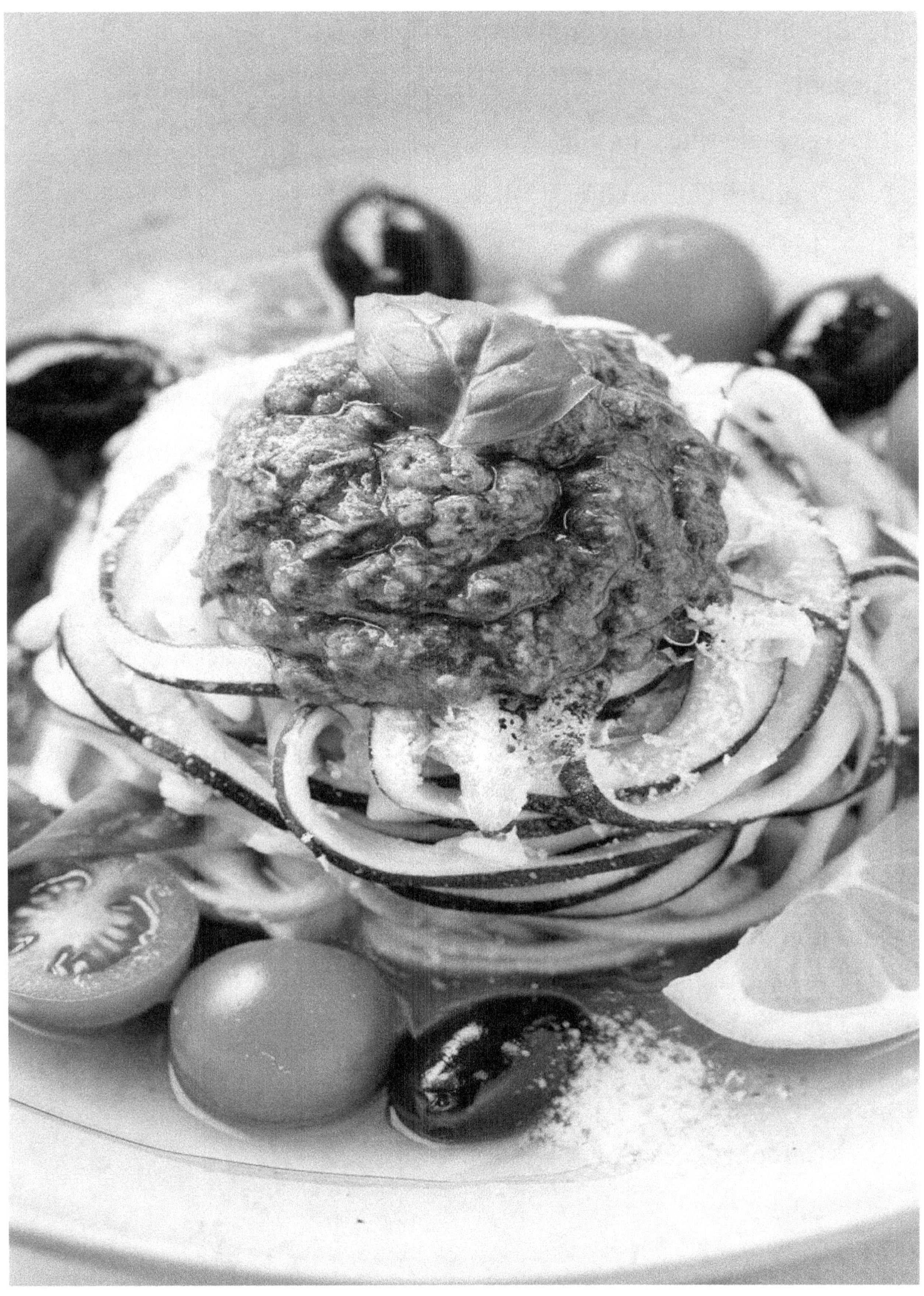

Recipe 8: Chicken Caesar Wrap

Ingredients:

- 1 whole wheat tortilla
- 1 grilled chicken breast, sliced
- 1 cup romaine lettuce, chopped
- 2 tbsp Caesar dressing
- ¼ cup Parmesan cheese, grated
- Optional: Croutons, black pepper

Instructions:

1. **Grill the Chicken:** Season chicken with salt and pepper, then grill until fully cooked. Slice into strips.

2. **Assemble the Wrap:** Place the tortilla on a flat surface. Layer with chopped romaine lettuce, grilled chicken, Caesar dressing, and Parmesan cheese.

3. **Fold and Roll:** Fold the sides of the tortilla inward, then roll up tightly.

4. **Serve:** Slice in half and serve with a side of fresh vegetables or fruit.

Nutritional Information (per serving):

- Calories: 400
- Protein: 30g
- Fat: 18g
- Carbohydrates: 35g
- Fiber: 7g

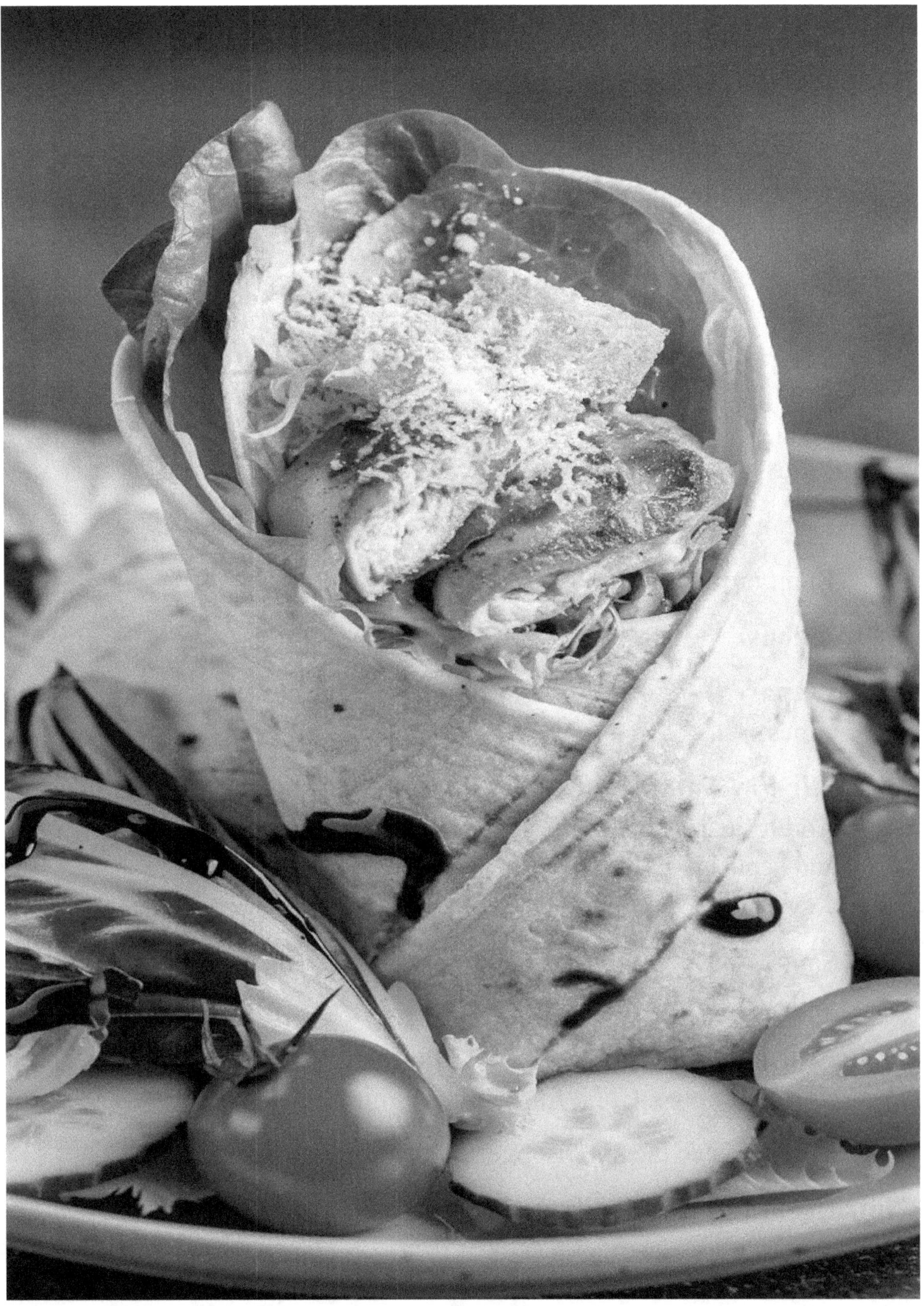

Recipe 9: Vegetable Stir-Fry with Tofu

Ingredients:

- 1 block firm tofu, drained and cubed
- 1 red bell pepper, sliced
- 1 cup broccoli florets
- 1 carrot, julienned
- 2 tbsp soy sauce (low sodium)
- 1 tbsp sesame oil
- 1 garlic clove, minced
- 1 tsp ginger, minced
- 1 cup brown rice, cooked

Instructions:

1. **Prepare the Tofu:** Press tofu to remove excess water, then cut into cubes.
2. **Stir-Fry Tofu:** Heat sesame oil in a large pan over medium heat. Add tofu and cook until golden on all sides. Remove from the pan and set aside.
3. **Cook the Vegetables:** In the same pan, add garlic and ginger. Sauté for 1 minute. Add bell pepper, broccoli, and carrot. Cook until vegetables are tender-crisp.
4. **Add Tofu and Sauce:** Return tofu to the pan, add soy sauce, and stir to combine. Cook for another 2 minutes.
5. **Serve:** Serve the stir-fry over cooked brown rice.

Nutritional Information (per serving):

- Calories: 350

- Protein: 15g

- Fat: 12g

- Carbohydrates: 45g

- Fiber: 8g

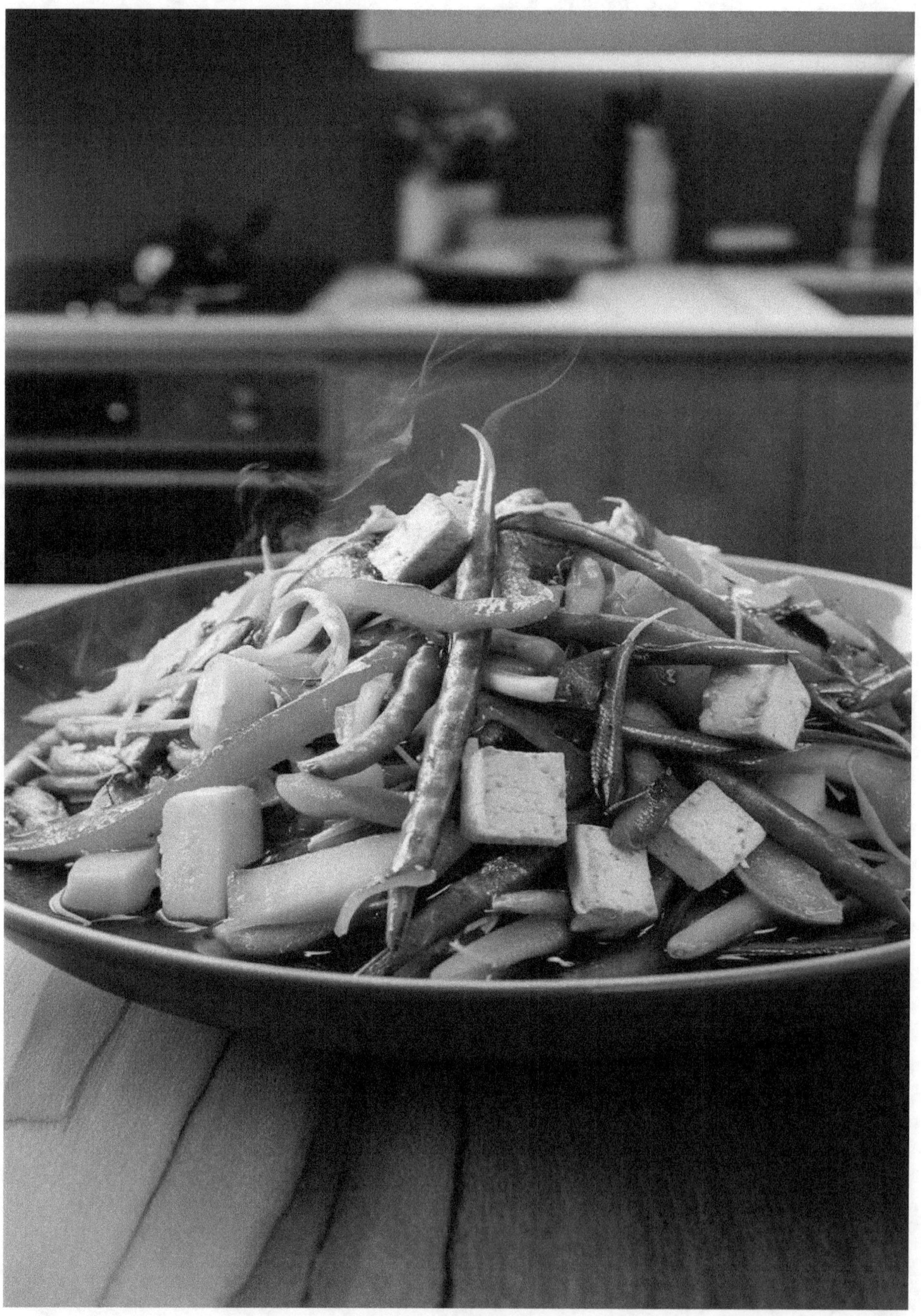

Recipe 10: Lentil Soup

Ingredients:

- 1 cup lentils, rinsed
- 1 carrot, diced
- 1 celery stalk, diced
- 1 onion, diced
- 2 garlic cloves, minced
- 4 cups vegetable broth
- 1 tsp cumin
- 1 tsp turmeric
- Salt and pepper to taste
- Optional: Fresh cilantro, lemon wedges

Instructions:

1. **Sauté Vegetables:** Heat a large pot over medium heat. Add diced onion, carrot, and celery. Cook until softened.
2. **Add Garlic and Spices:** Stir in minced garlic, cumin, and turmeric. Cook for 1 minute until fragrant.
3. **Add Lentils and Broth:** Pour in lentils and vegetable broth. Bring to a boil, then reduce heat to low. Simmer for 20-25 minutes until lentils are tender.
4. **Season:** Season with salt and pepper to taste.
5. **Serve:** Ladle the soup into bowls and garnish with fresh cilantro and a squeeze of lemon juice if desired.

Nutritional Information (per serving):

- Calories: 250

- Fat: 3g

- Carbohydrates: 45g

- Fiber: 15g

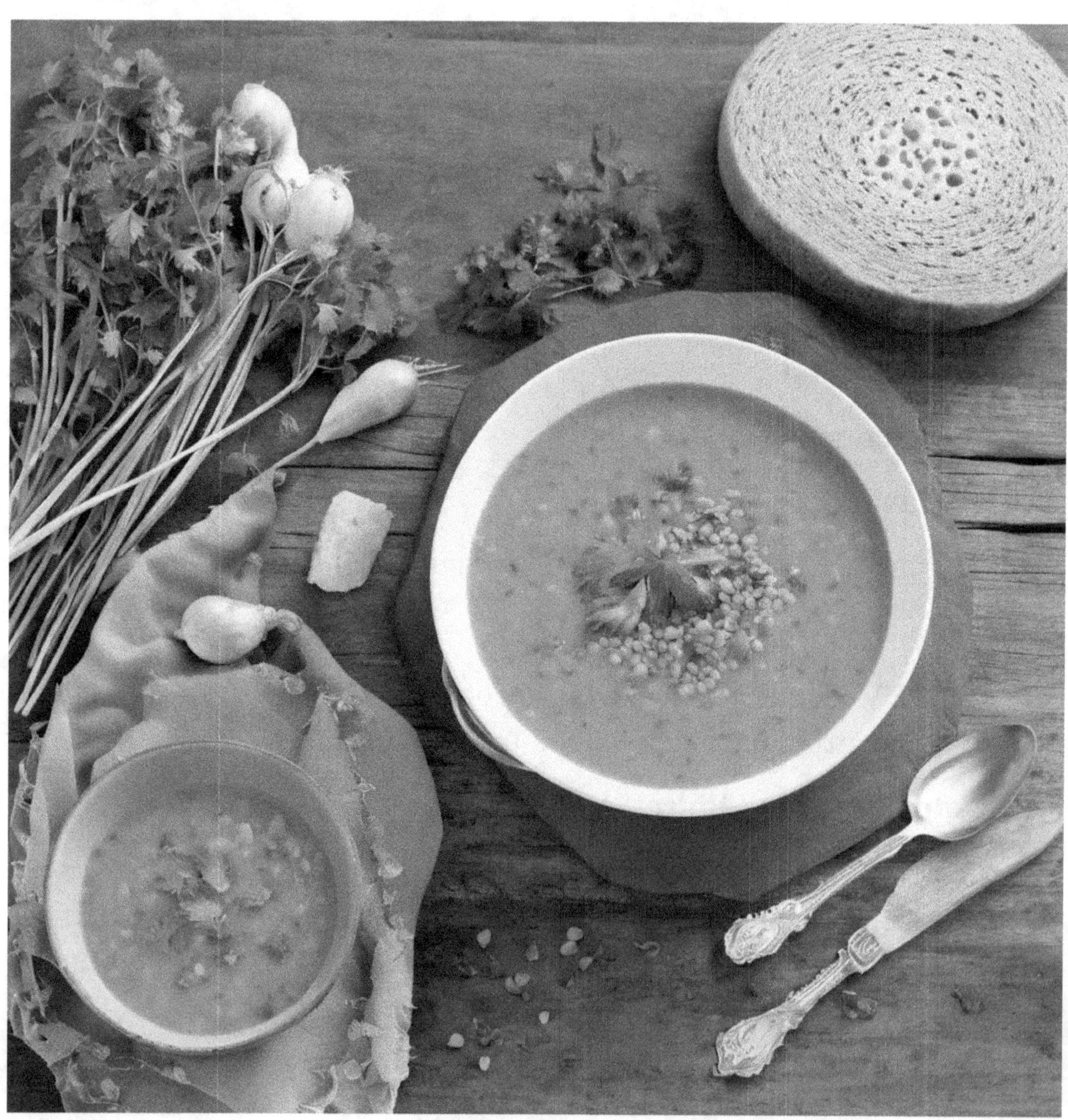

Dinner Recipes

Recipe 11: Grilled Salmon with Asparagus

Ingredients:

- 1 salmon fillet
- 1 bunch asparagus, trimmed
- 2 tbsp olive oil
- 1 lemon, sliced
- 1 tsp fresh dill, chopped
- Salt and pepper to taste

Instructions:

1. **Preheat the Grill:** Preheat your grill to medium-high heat.
2. **Season the Salmon:** Drizzle the salmon fillet with 1 tbsp olive oil and season with salt, pepper, and dill.
3. **Grill the Salmon:** Place the salmon on the grill, skin side down. Grill for 6-8 minutes on each side until the fish flakes easily with a fork.
4. **Prepare the Asparagus:** Toss asparagus with remaining olive oil, salt, and pepper.
5. **Grill the Asparagus:** Grill asparagus for 4-5 minutes, turning occasionally, until tender and slightly charred.
6. **Serve:** Plate the grilled salmon with asparagus and garnish with lemon slices.

Nutritional Information (per serving):

- Calories: 350
- Protein: 30g
- Fat: 20g
- Carbohydrates: 5g
- Fiber: 3g

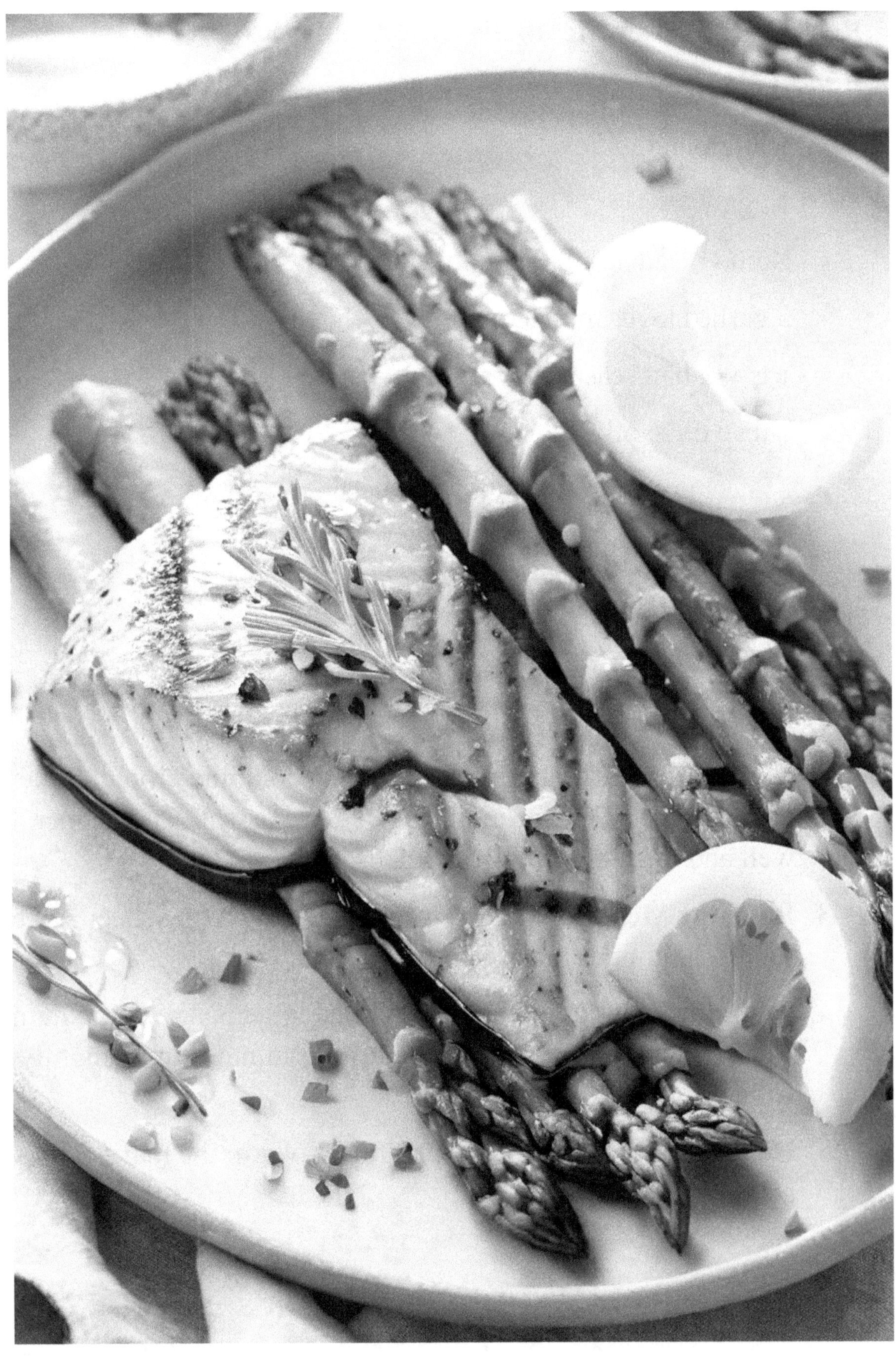

Recipe 12: Turkey Meatballs with Zoodles

Ingredients:

- 1 lb ground turkey
- 1 egg
- ½ cup breadcrumbs (whole wheat)
- 2 garlic cloves, minced
- 1 tsp Italian seasoning
- 1 tbsp olive oil
- 2 zucchinis, spiralized into noodles
- 2 cups marinara sauce
- Optional: Parmesan cheese, fresh basil

Instructions:

1. **Preheat the Oven:** Preheat your oven to 400°F (200°C).
2. **Make the Meatballs:** In a large bowl, combine ground turkey, egg, breadcrumbs, garlic, Italian seasoning, salt, and pepper. Mix well and form into small meatballs.
3. **Bake the Meatballs:** Place meatballs on a baking sheet and bake for 15-20 minutes until cooked through.
4. **Cook the Zoodles:** Heat olive oil in a large pan over medium heat. Add zucchini noodles and sauté for 2-3 minutes until slightly softened.
5. **Heat the Marinara:** In a separate pot, warm the marinara sauce over low heat.

6. **Assemble the Dish:** Serve meatballs over zoodles, topped with marinara sauce. Garnish with Parmesan cheese and fresh basil if desired.

Nutritional Information (per serving):

- Calories: 400
- Protein: 35g
- Fat: 18g
- Carbohydrates: 20g
- Fiber: 5g

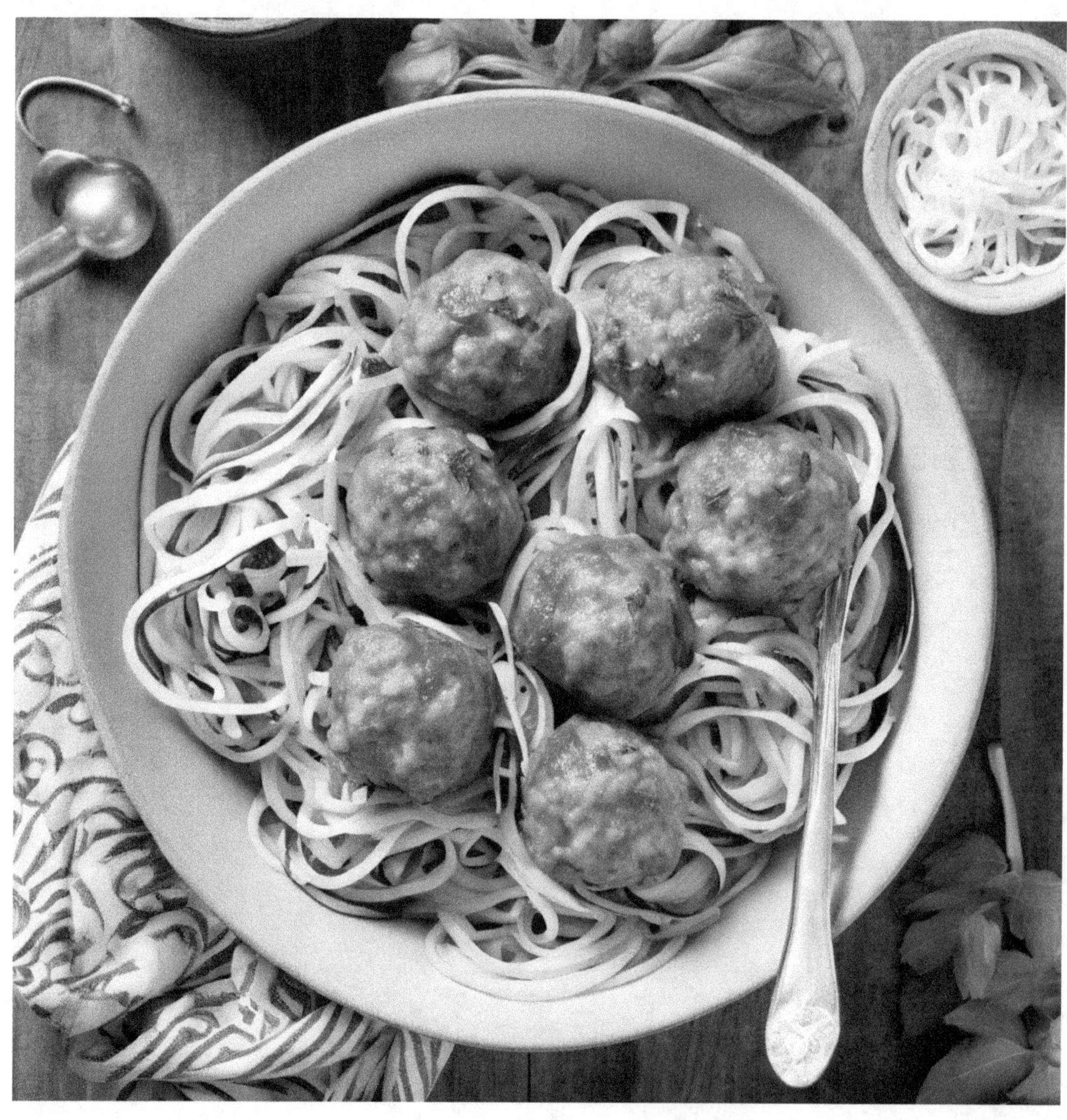

Recipe 13: Stuffed Bell Peppers

Ingredients:

- 4 bell peppers (any color), tops cut off and seeds removed
- 1 cup cooked quinoa
- 1 can black beans, drained and rinsed
- ½ cup corn kernels (fresh or frozen)
- 1 cup shredded cheese (cheddar or mozzarella)
- 1 cup salsa
- Optional: Fresh cilantro, avocado

Instructions:

1. **Preheat the Oven:** Preheat your oven to 375°F (190°C).
2. **Prepare the Filling:** In a large bowl, combine cooked quinoa, black beans, corn, ½ cup shredded cheese, and salsa. Mix well.
3. **Stuff the Peppers:** Spoon the filling into each bell pepper, packing it tightly.
4. **Bake:** Place the stuffed peppers in a baking dish. Cover with foil and bake for 30 minutes. Remove the foil, top with remaining cheese, and bake for an additional 10 minutes until the cheese is melted and bubbly.
5. **Serve:** Garnish with fresh cilantro and avocado slices if desired.

Nutritional Information (per serving):

- Calories: 350
- Protein: 15g
- Fat: 12g
- Carbohydrates: 45g
- Fiber: 10g

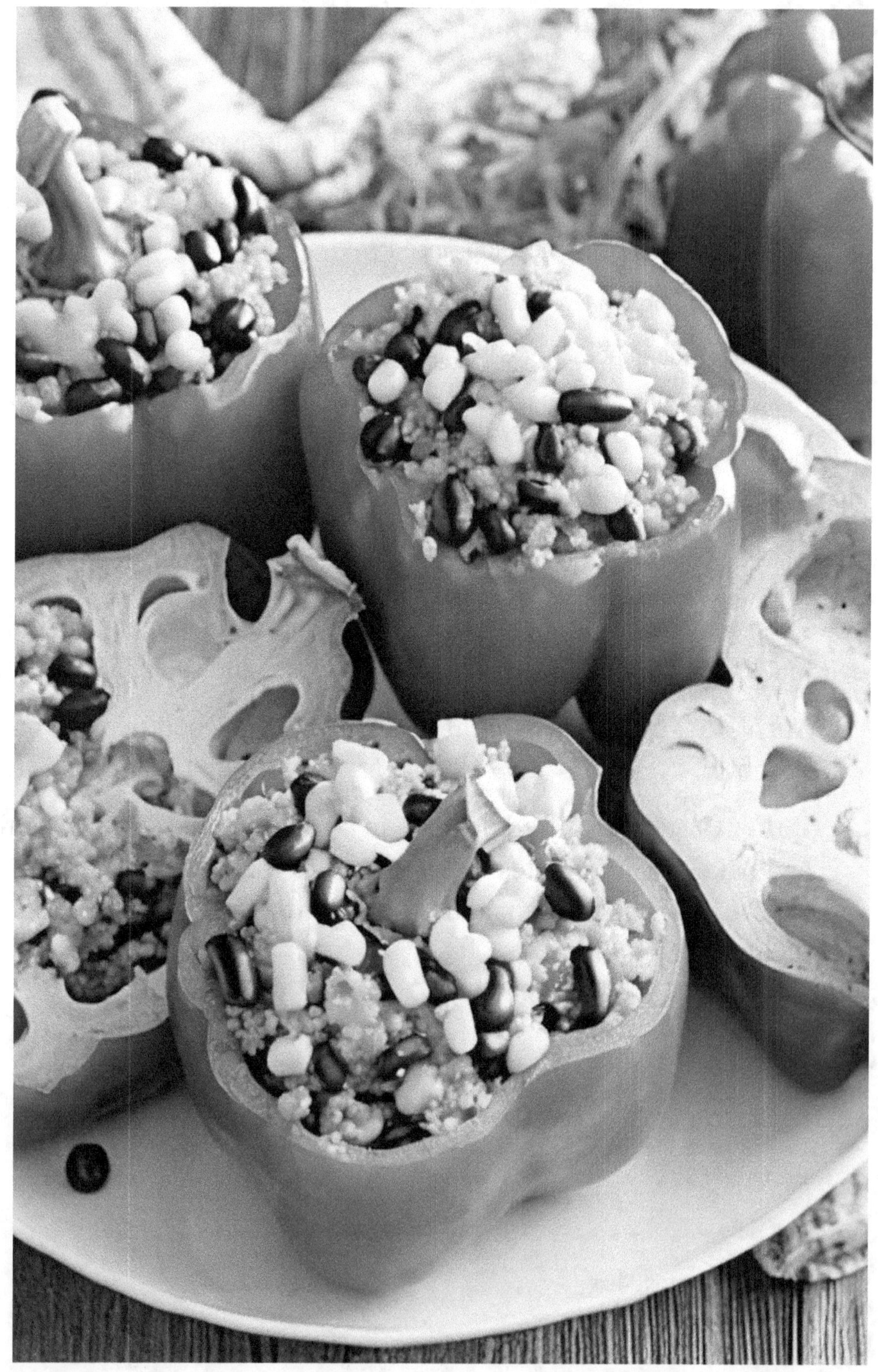

Recipe 14: Baked Cod with Sweet Potatoes

Ingredients:

- 2 cod fillets
- 2 medium sweet potatoes, peeled and cubed
- 2 tbsp olive oil
- 2 garlic cloves, minced
- 1 tsp fresh thyme, chopped
- 1 lemon, sliced
- Salt and pepper to taste

Instructions:

1. **Preheat the Oven:** Preheat your oven to 400°F (200°C).
2. **Roast the Sweet Potatoes:** Toss sweet potatoes with 1 tbsp olive oil, garlic, thyme, salt, and pepper. Spread on a baking sheet and roast for 20-25 minutes until tender.
3. **Bake the Cod:** Season cod fillets with salt and pepper. Place on a baking sheet, drizzle with remaining olive oil, and top with lemon slices. Bake for 12-15 minutes until the fish flakes easily with a fork.
4. **Serve:** Plate the baked cod with roasted sweet potatoes on the side.

Nutritional Information (per serving):

- Calories: 350
- Protein: 25g
- Fat: 12g
- Carbohydrates: 40g
- Fiber: 8g

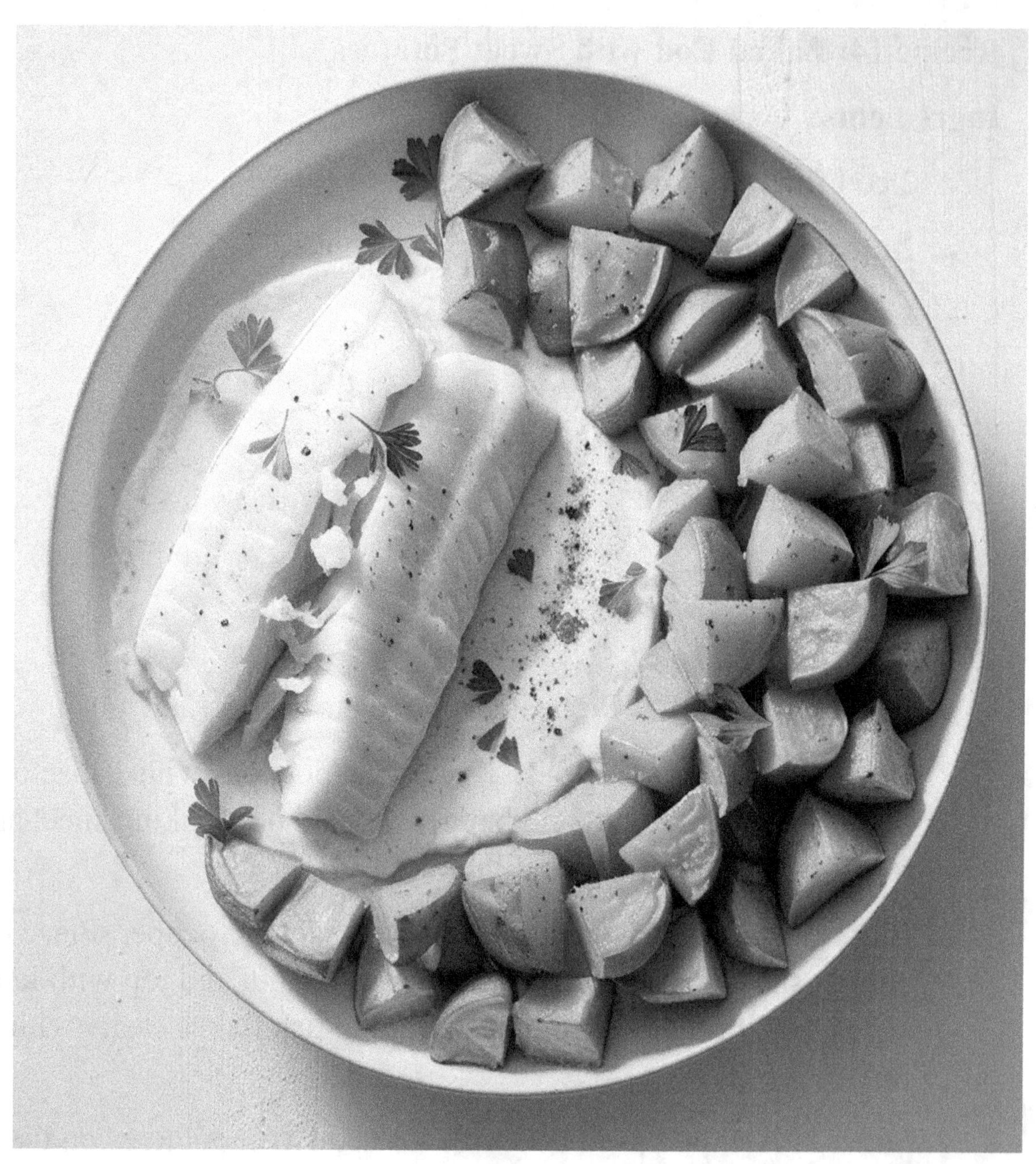

Recipe 15: Vegetable Curry with Brown Rice

Ingredients:

- 1 tbsp coconut oil
- 1 onion, diced
- 2 garlic cloves, minced
- 1 tbsp curry powder
- 1 tsp turmeric
- 1 tsp cumin
- 1 can coconut milk (light)
- 2 cups mixed vegetables (e.g., bell peppers, carrots, peas)
- 1 can chickpeas, drained and rinsed
- 1 cup brown rice, cooked
- Optional: Fresh cilantro, lime wedges

Instructions:

1. **Sauté the Onion:** Heat coconut oil in a large pot over medium heat. Add diced onion and cook until softened.
2. **Add Garlic and Spices:** Stir in minced garlic, curry powder, turmeric, and cumin. Cook for 1-2 minutes until fragrant.
3. **Add Vegetables and Coconut Milk:** Add mixed vegetables, chickpeas, and coconut milk to the pot. Bring to a simmer and cook for 10-15 minutes until vegetables are tender.
4. **Serve:** Serve the curry over cooked brown rice. Garnish with fresh cilantro and a squeeze of lime juice if desired.

Nutritional Information (per serving):

- Calories: 400

- Protein: 12g
- Fat: 18g
- Carbohydrates: 55g
- Fiber: 10g

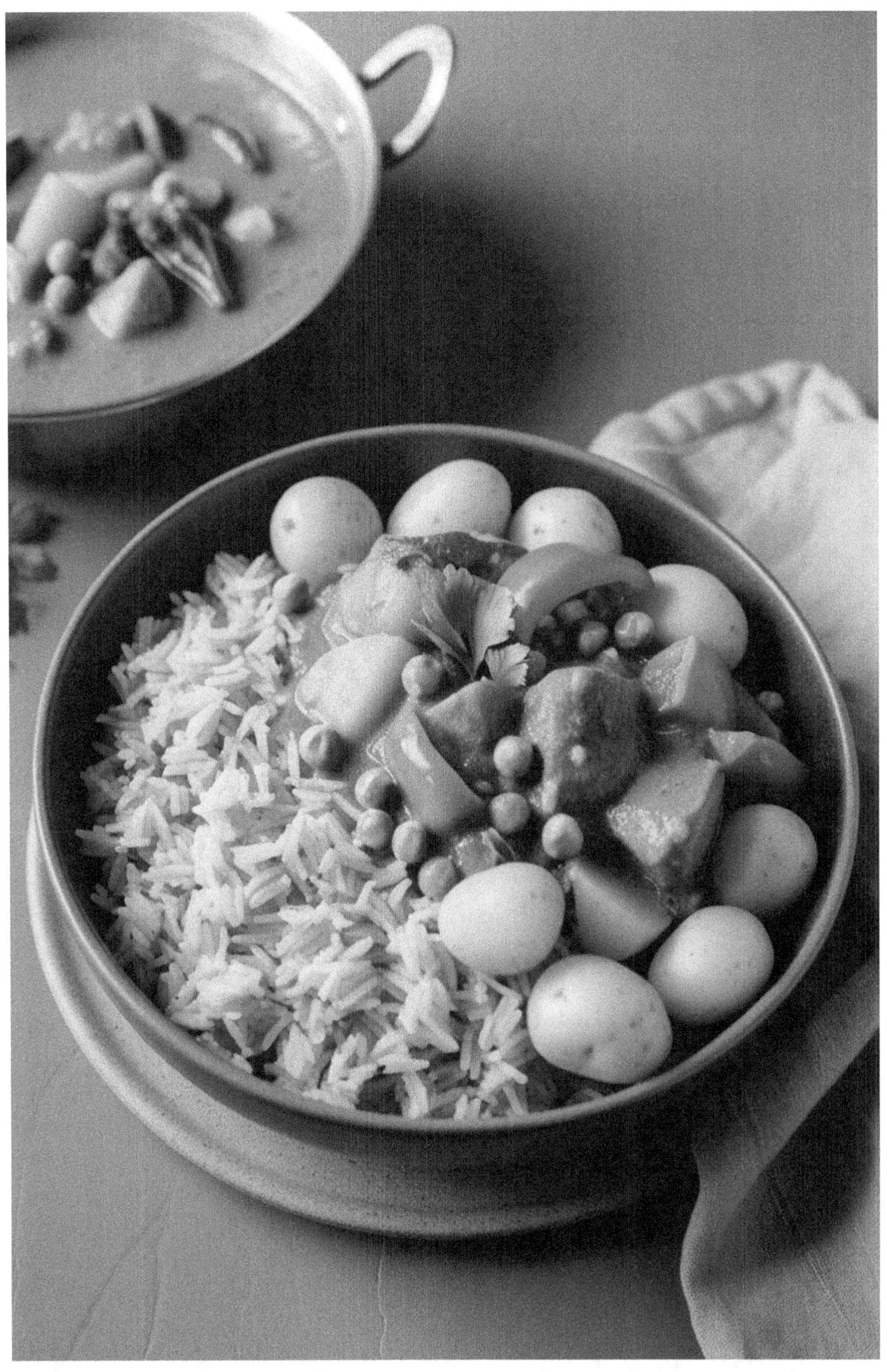

Snack Recipes

Recipe 16: Hummus with Veggie Sticks

Ingredients:

- 1 can chickpeas, drained and rinsed
- 2 tbsp tahini
- 2 tbsp olive oil
- 1 garlic clove, minced
- 1 lemon, juiced
- Salt and pepper to taste
- Veggie sticks (carrots, celery, bell peppers, cucumber)

Instructions:

1. **Blend the Hummus:** In a food processor, combine chickpeas, tahini, olive oil, garlic, lemon juice, salt, and pepper. Blend until smooth. Add water if needed to reach desired consistency.

2. **Serve:** Transfer hummus to a bowl and serve with assorted veggie sticks.

Nutritional Information (per serving):

- Calories: 200
- Protein: 6g
- Fat: 12g
- Carbohydrates: 20g
- Fiber: 6g

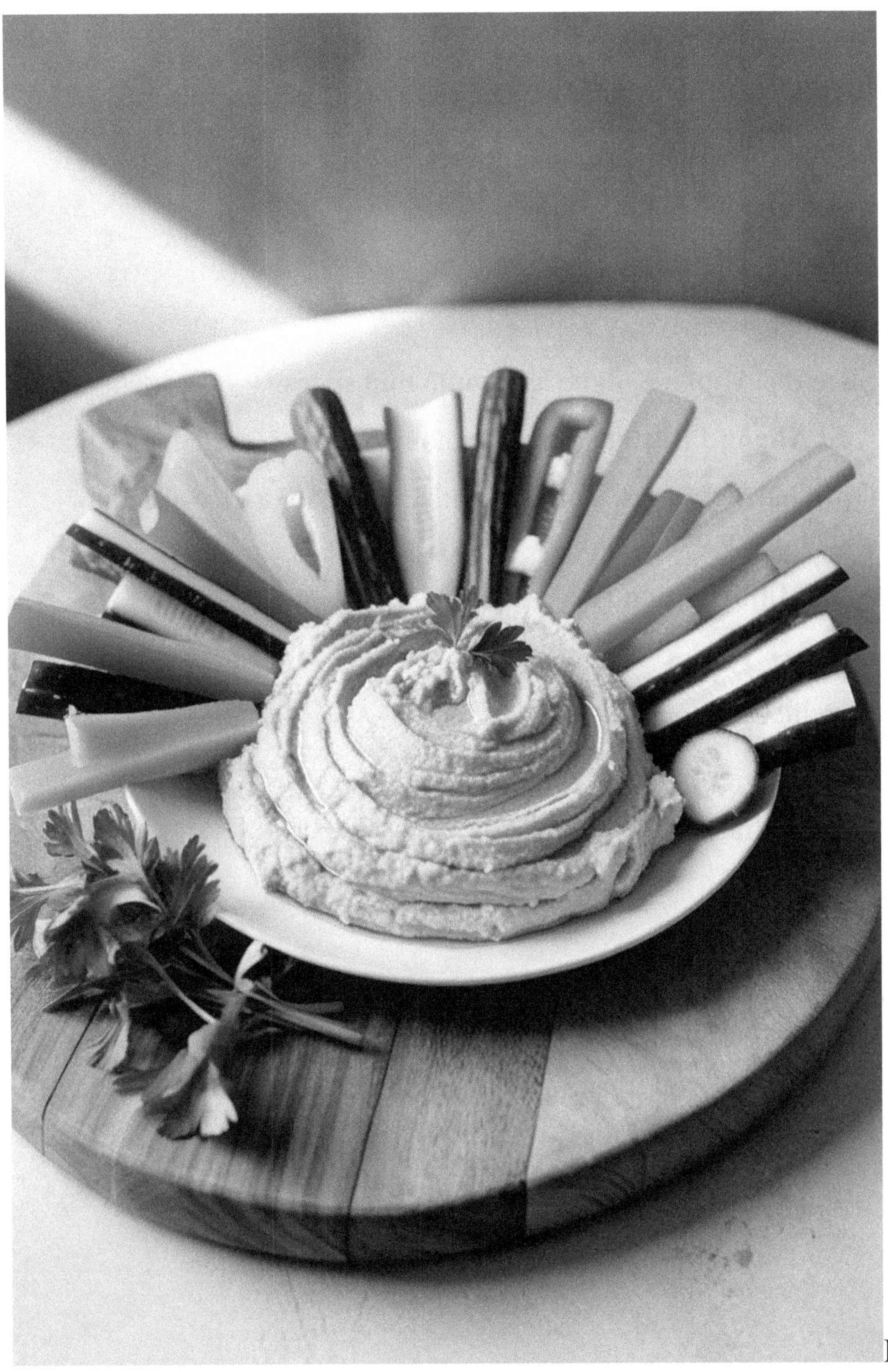

pe 17: Apple Slices with Almond Butter

Ingredients:

- 1 apple, sliced
- 2 tbsp almond butter
- Optional: Cinnamon, chia seeds

Instructions:

1. **Slice the Apple:** Cut the apple into thin slices.
2. **Add Almond Butter:** Spread almond butter on each apple slice.
3. **Optional Toppings:** Sprinkle with cinnamon or chia seeds for added flavor and texture.

Nutritional Information (per serving):

- Calories: 250
- Protein: 5g
- Fat: 15g
- Carbohydrates: 25g
- Fiber: 8g

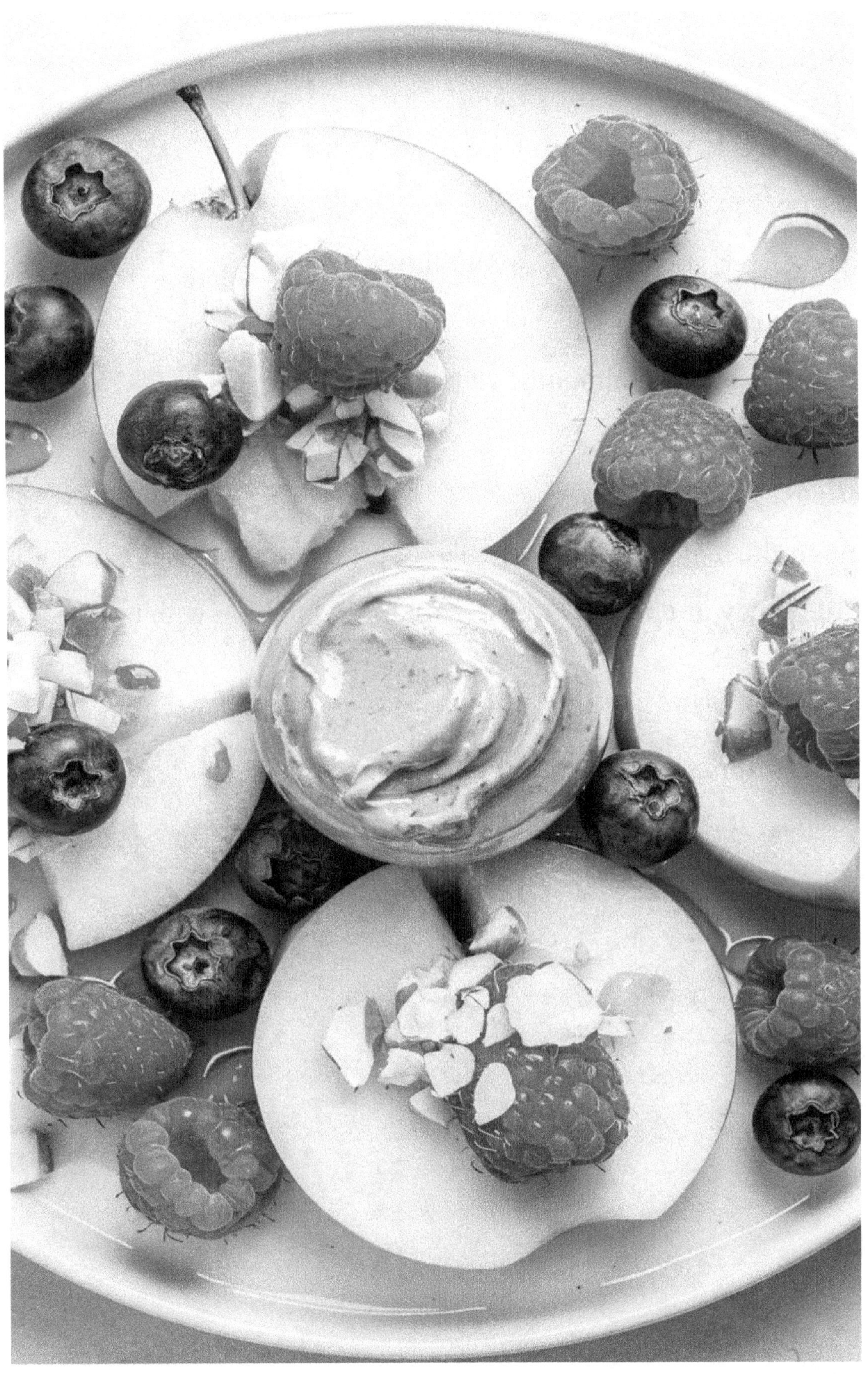

Recipe 18: Greek Yogurt with Honey and Nuts

Ingredients:

- 1 cup Greek yogurt (plain or vanilla)
- 1 tbsp honey
- ¼ cup mixed nuts (almonds, walnuts, pecans)
- Optional: Fresh fruit

Instructions:

1. **Spoon the Yogurt:** Spoon Greek yogurt into a bowl.
2. **Add Honey and Nuts:** Drizzle with honey and top with mixed nuts.
3. **Optional:** Add fresh fruit for added sweetness and nutrition.

Nutritional Information (per serving):

- Calories: 300
- Protein: 15g
- Fat: 15g
- Carbohydrates: 25g
- Fiber: 4g

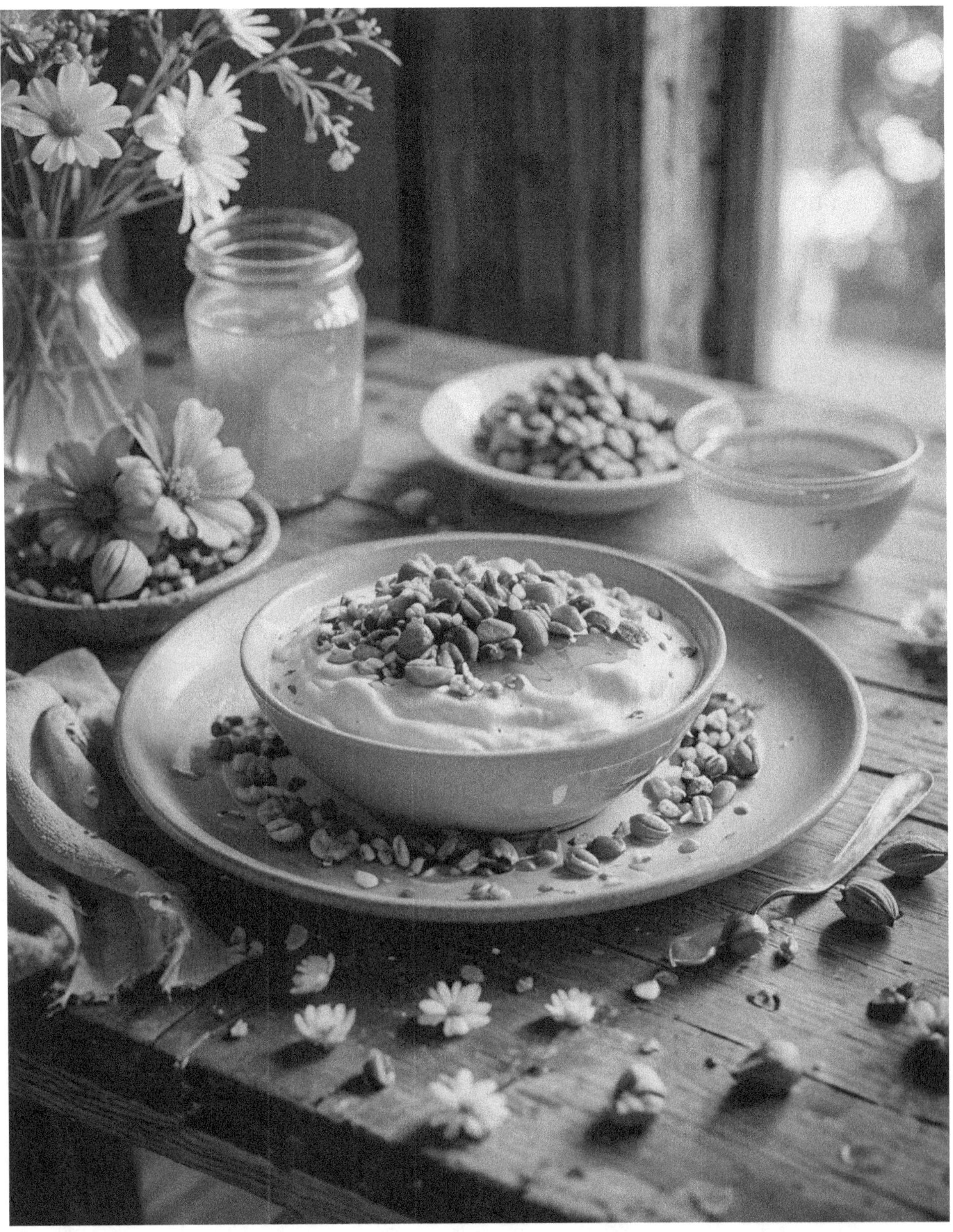

Recipe 19: Energy Balls

Ingredients:

- 1 cup oats
- ½ cup peanut butter (or any nut butter)
- ¼ cup honey
- ¼ cup flax seeds
- ¼ cup chocolate chips (optional)
- 1 tsp vanilla extract

Instructions:

1. **Mix the Ingredients:** In a large bowl, combine oats, peanut butter, honey, flax seeds, chocolate chips, and vanilla extract. Mix until well combined.
2. **Form Balls:** Roll the mixture into small balls using your hands. Place on a baking sheet lined with parchment paper.
3. **Refrigerate:** Refrigerate for at least 30 minutes to set.
4. **Serve:** Store in an airtight container in the fridge for up to a week.

Nutritional Information (per serving, 2 balls):

- Calories: 200
- Protein: 6g
- Fat: 10g
- Carbohydrates: 25g
- Fiber: 4g

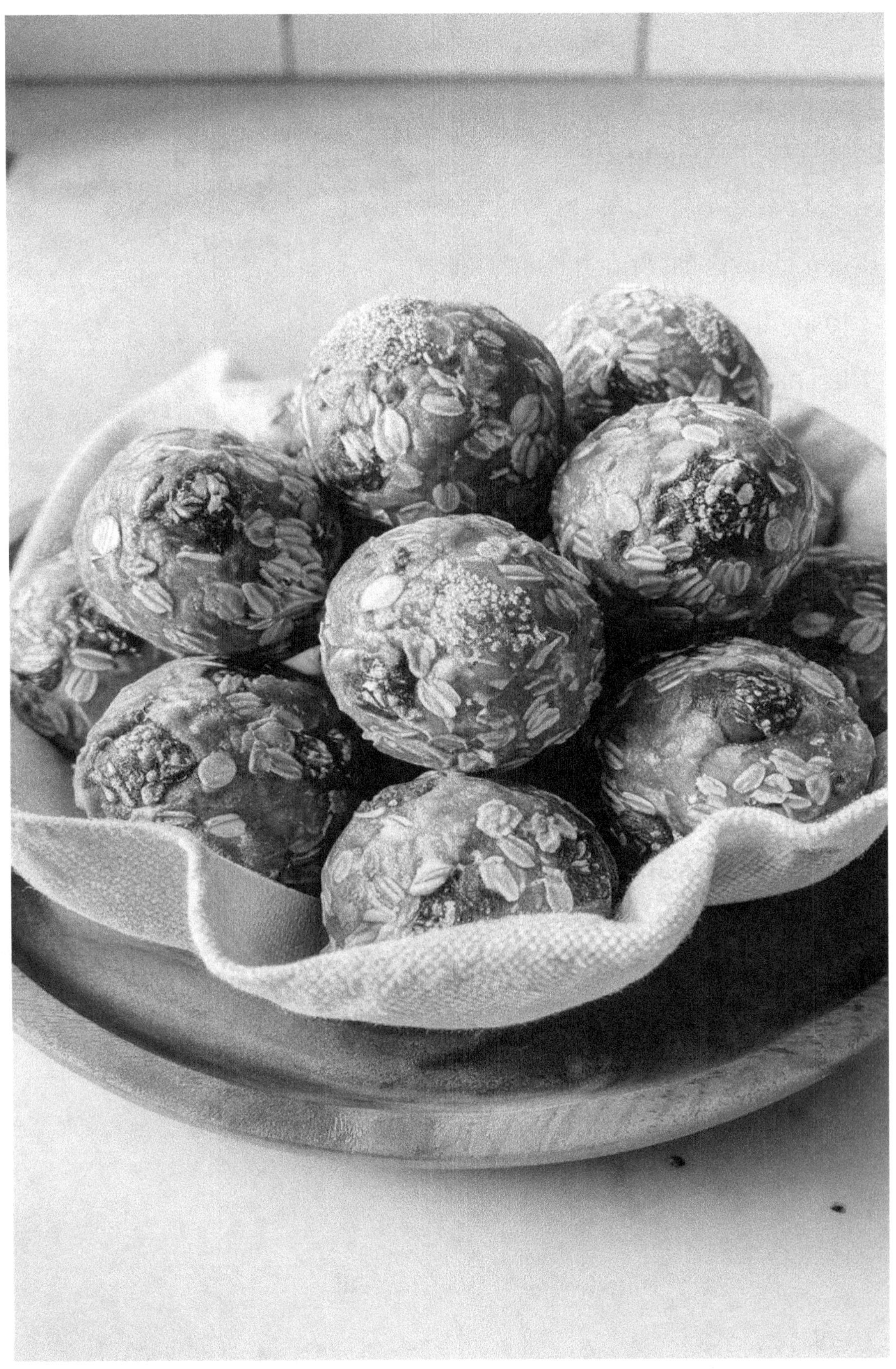

Recipe 20: Roasted Chickpeas

Ingredients:

- 1 can chickpeas, drained and rinsed
- 1 tbsp olive oil
- 1 tsp paprika
- 1 tsp cumin
- Salt and pepper to taste

Instructions:

1. **Preheat the Oven:** Preheat your oven to 400°F (200°C).
2. **Prepare the Chickpeas:** Pat chickpeas dry with a paper towel. Toss with olive oil, paprika, cumin, salt, and pepper.
3. **Roast:** Spread chickpeas on a baking sheet and roast for 20-25 minutes until crispy.
4. **Serve:** Let cool slightly before serving as a crunchy snack.

Nutritional Information (per serving):

- Calories: 150
- Protein: 6g
- Fat: 6g
- Carbohydrates: 18g
- Fiber: 6g

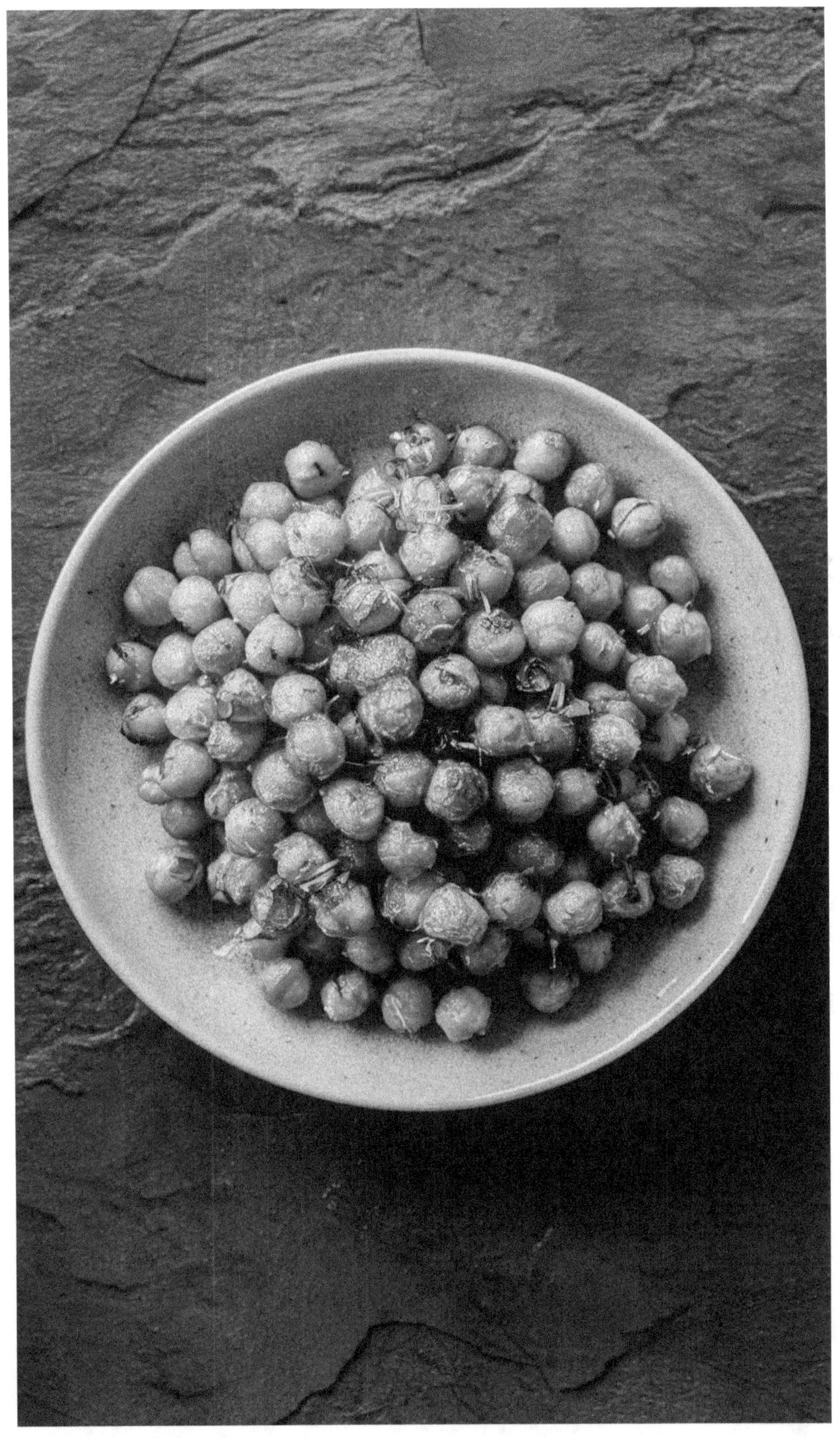

Dessert Recipes

Recipe 21: Chia Seed Pudding

Ingredients:

- ¼ cup chia seeds
- 1 cup almond milk (or any milk of choice)
- 1 tbsp honey or maple syrup
- 1 tsp vanilla extract
- Optional toppings: Fresh fruit, nuts, coconut flakes

Instructions:

1. **Mix Ingredients:** In a bowl or mason jar, combine chia seeds, milk, honey, and vanilla extract. Stir well.
2. **Refrigerate:** Cover and refrigerate for at least 4 hours or overnight until the pudding thickens.
3. **Add Toppings:** Before serving, stir the pudding and top with fresh fruit, nuts, or coconut flakes.

Nutritional Information (per serving):

- Calories: 200
- Protein: 6g
- Fat: 12g
- Carbohydrates: 18g
- Fiber: 10g

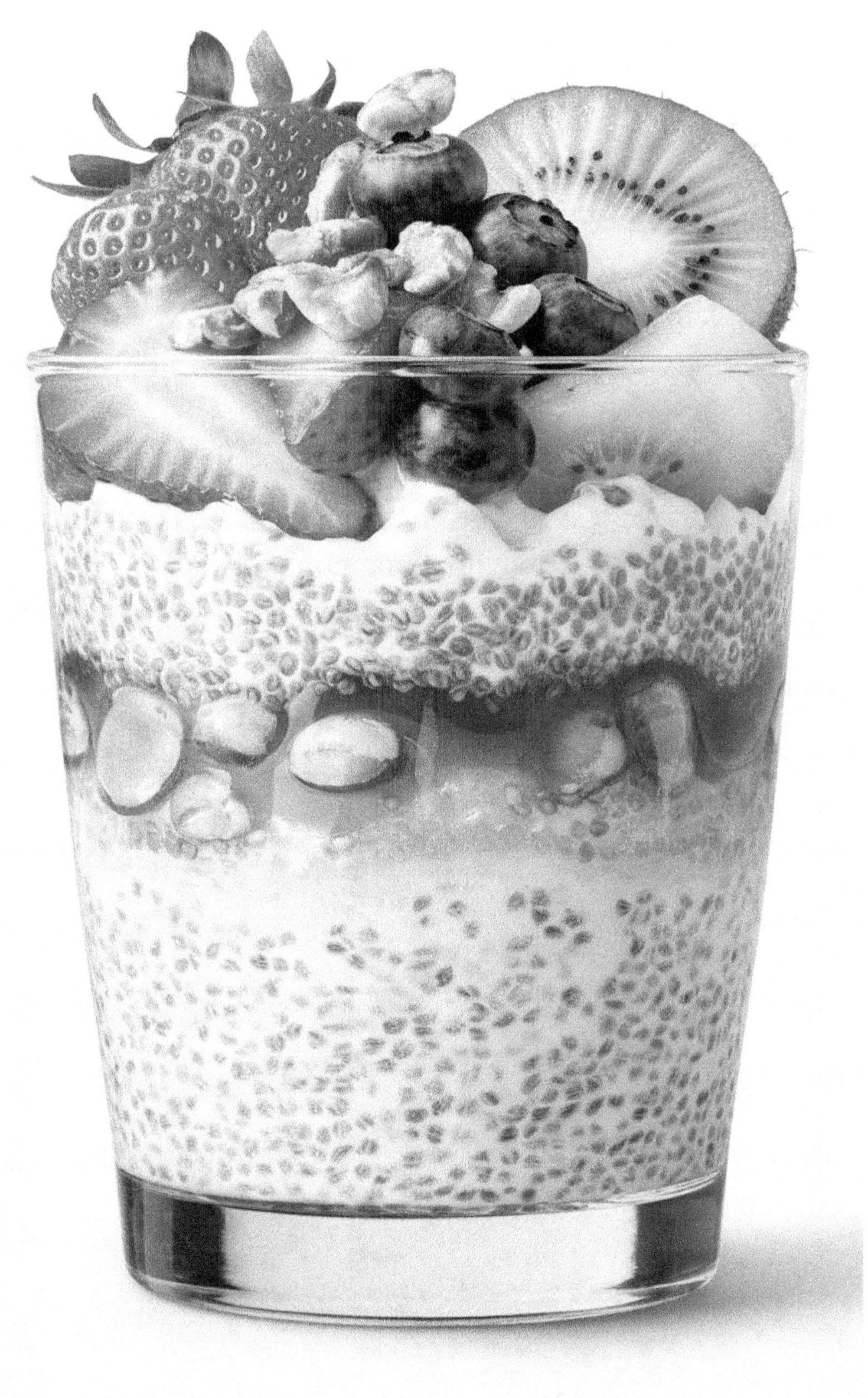

Recipe 22: Baked Apples with Cinnamon

Ingredients:

- 2 apples, cored and sliced
- 1 tbsp honey
- 1 tsp cinnamon
- ¼ cup oats
- Optional: Nuts, raisins

Instructions:

1. **Preheat the Oven:** Preheat your oven to 350°F (175°C).
2. **Prepare the Apples:** Place sliced apples in a baking dish. Drizzle with honey and sprinkle with cinnamon and oats.
3. **Bake:** Bake for 20-25 minutes until apples are tender.
4. **Serve:** Serve warm, optionally topped with nuts or raisins.

Nutritional Information (per serving):

- Calories: 150
- Protein: 2g
- Fat: 3g
- Carbohydrates: 30g
- Fiber: 5g

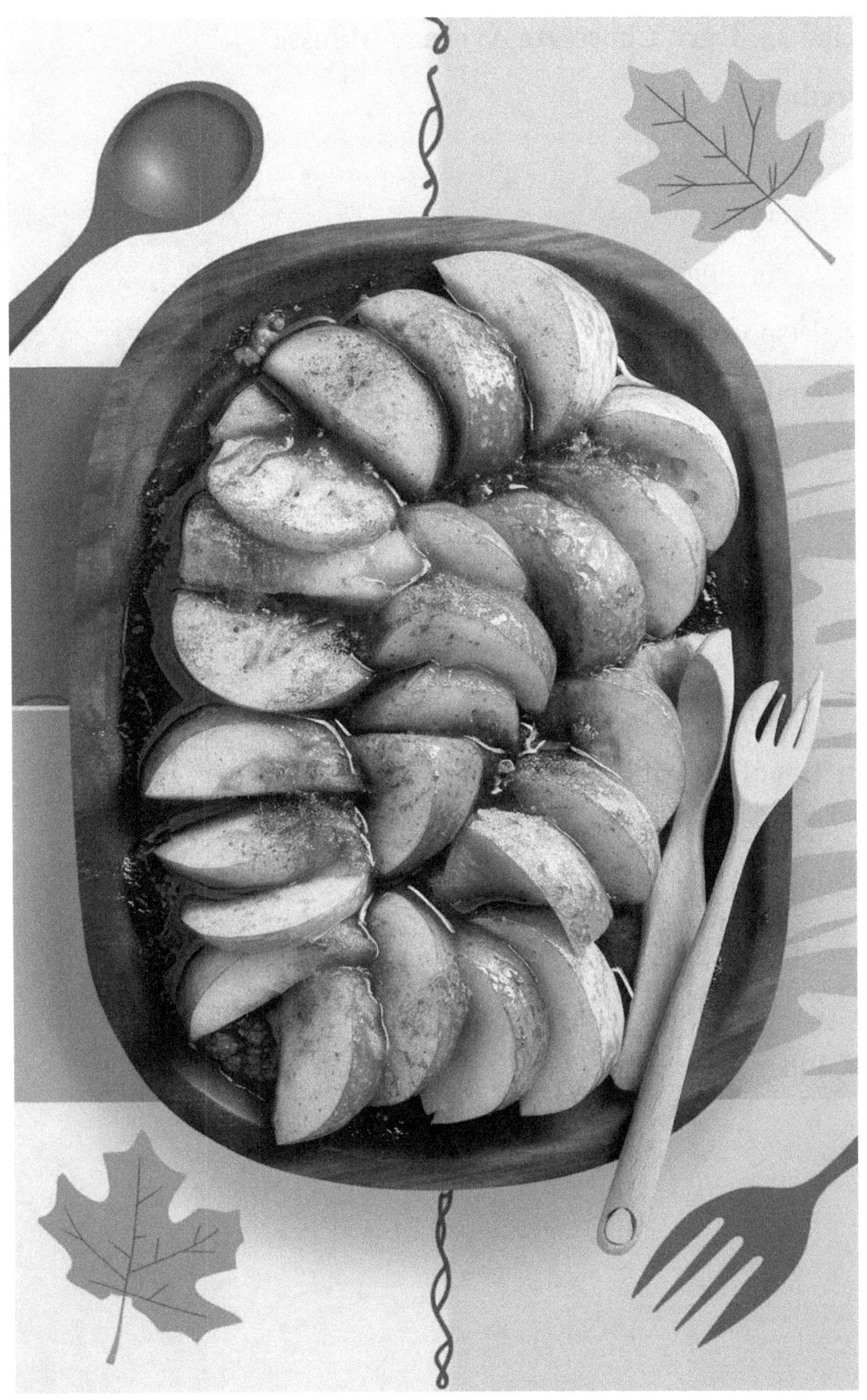

Recipe 23: Dark Chocolate Avocado Mousse

Ingredients:

- 2 ripe avocados
- ¼ cup cocoa powder
- ¼ cup honey or maple syrup
- 1 tsp vanilla extract
- Optional: Berries, mint leaves

Instructions:

1. **Blend Ingredients:** In a food processor, blend avocados, cocoa powder, honey, and vanilla extract until smooth and creamy.
2. **Chill:** Refrigerate for at least 1 hour to allow the flavors to meld.
3. **Serve:** Spoon mousse into bowls and garnish with fresh berries or mint leaves.

Nutritional Information (per serving):

- Calories: 250
- Protein: 3g
- Fat: 18g
- Carbohydrates: 24g
- Fiber: 10g

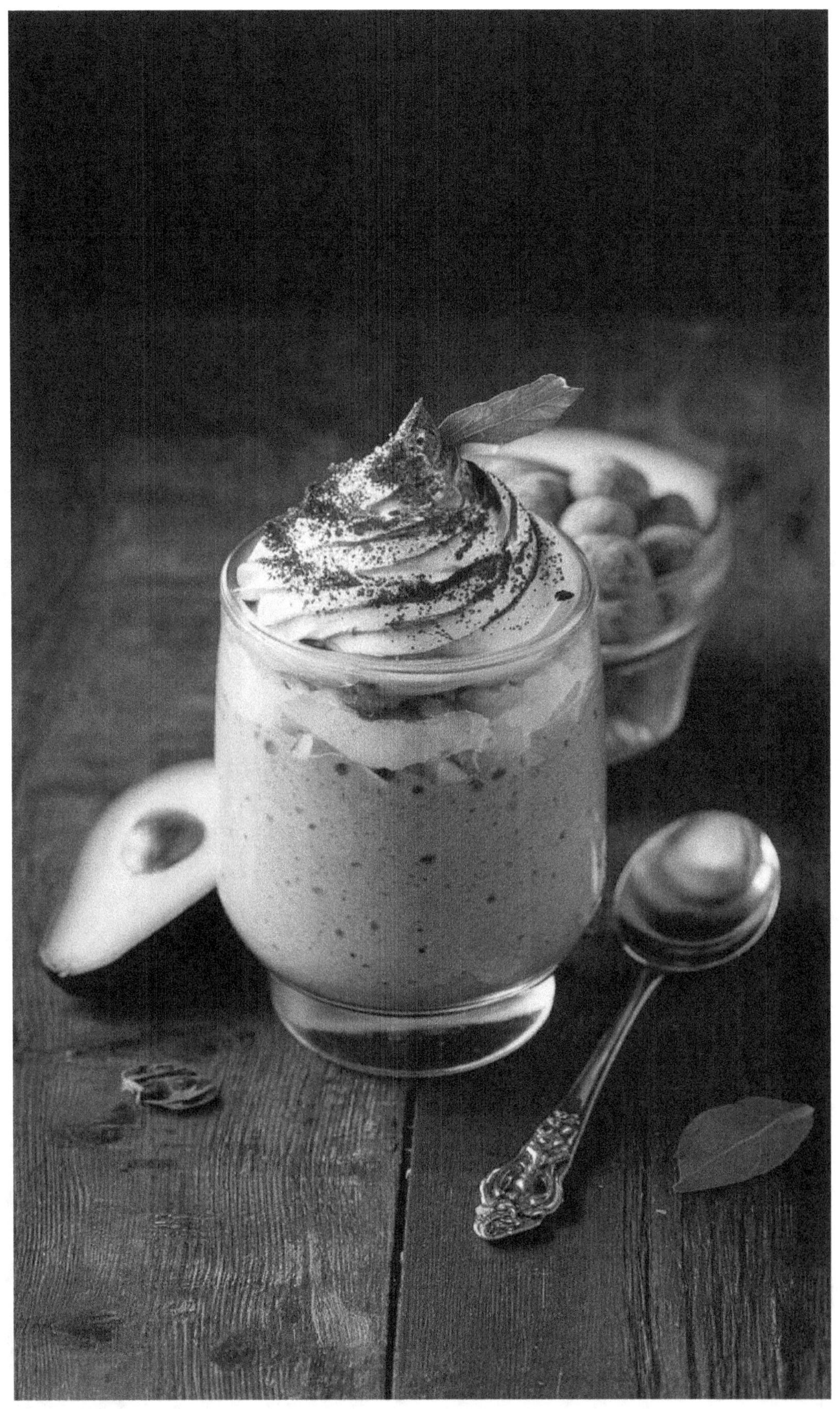

Recipe 24: Banana Nice Cream

Ingredients:

- 2 ripe bananas, sliced and frozen
- 1 tbsp almond butter
- 1 tsp vanilla extract
- Optional: Cocoa powder, berries, nuts

Instructions:

1. **Blend Bananas:** In a blender, combine frozen banana slices, almond butter, and vanilla extract. Blend until smooth and creamy, similar to soft-serve ice cream.
2. **Serve:** Serve immediately as a healthy alternative to ice cream, optionally topped with cocoa powder, berries, or nuts.

Ingredients:

- 2 cups rolled oats
- 1 cup almond milk
- 1 egg
- ¼ cup honey
- 1 tsp vanilla extract
- 1 tsp baking powder
- ½ cup mixed berries
- Optional: Nuts, chocolate chips

Instructions:

1. **Preheat the Oven:** Preheat your oven to 350°F (175°C).

2. **Mix the Ingredients:** In a large bowl, combine rolled oats, almond milk, egg, honey, vanilla extract, and baking powder. Stir in mixed berries.

3. **Bake:** Pour the mixture into a greased muffin tin, filling each cup about ¾ full. Bake for 20-25 minutes until golden brown.

4. **Serve:** Let cool slightly before removing from the muffin tin. Enjoy as a portable breakfast or snack.

Nutritional Information (per serving, 1 cup):

- Calories: 120

- Protein: 3g

- Fat: 3g

- Carbohydrates: 20g

- Fiber: 3g

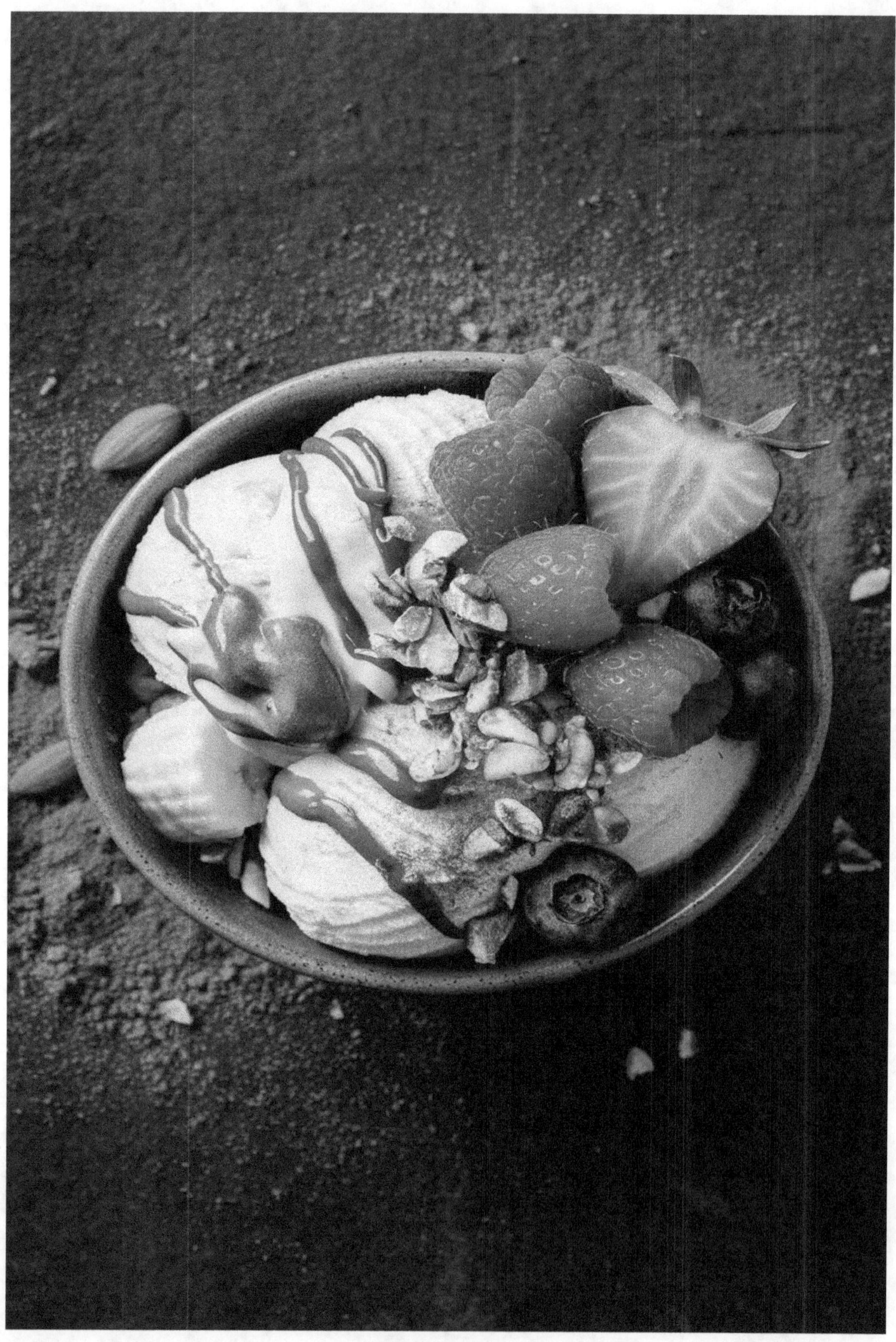

Recipe 25: Baked Oatmeal Cups

Ingredients:

- 2 cups rolled oats
- 1 cup almond milk
- 1 egg
- ¼ cup honey
- 1 tsp vanilla extract
- 1 tsp baking powder
- ½ cup mixed berries
- Optional: Nuts, chocolate chips

Instructions:

1. **Preheat the Oven:** Preheat your oven to 350°F (175°C).
2. **Mix the Ingredients:** In a large bowl, combine rolled oats, almond milk, egg, honey, vanilla extract, and baking powder. Stir in mixed berries.
3. **Bake:** Pour the mixture into a greased muffin tin, filling each cup about ¾ full. Bake for 20-25 minutes until golden brown.
4. **Serve:** Let cool slightly before removing from the muffin tin. Enjoy as a portable breakfast or snack.

Nutritional Information (per serving, 1 cup):

- Calories: 120
- Protein: 3g
- Fat: 3g
- Carbohydrates: 20g
- Fiber: 3g

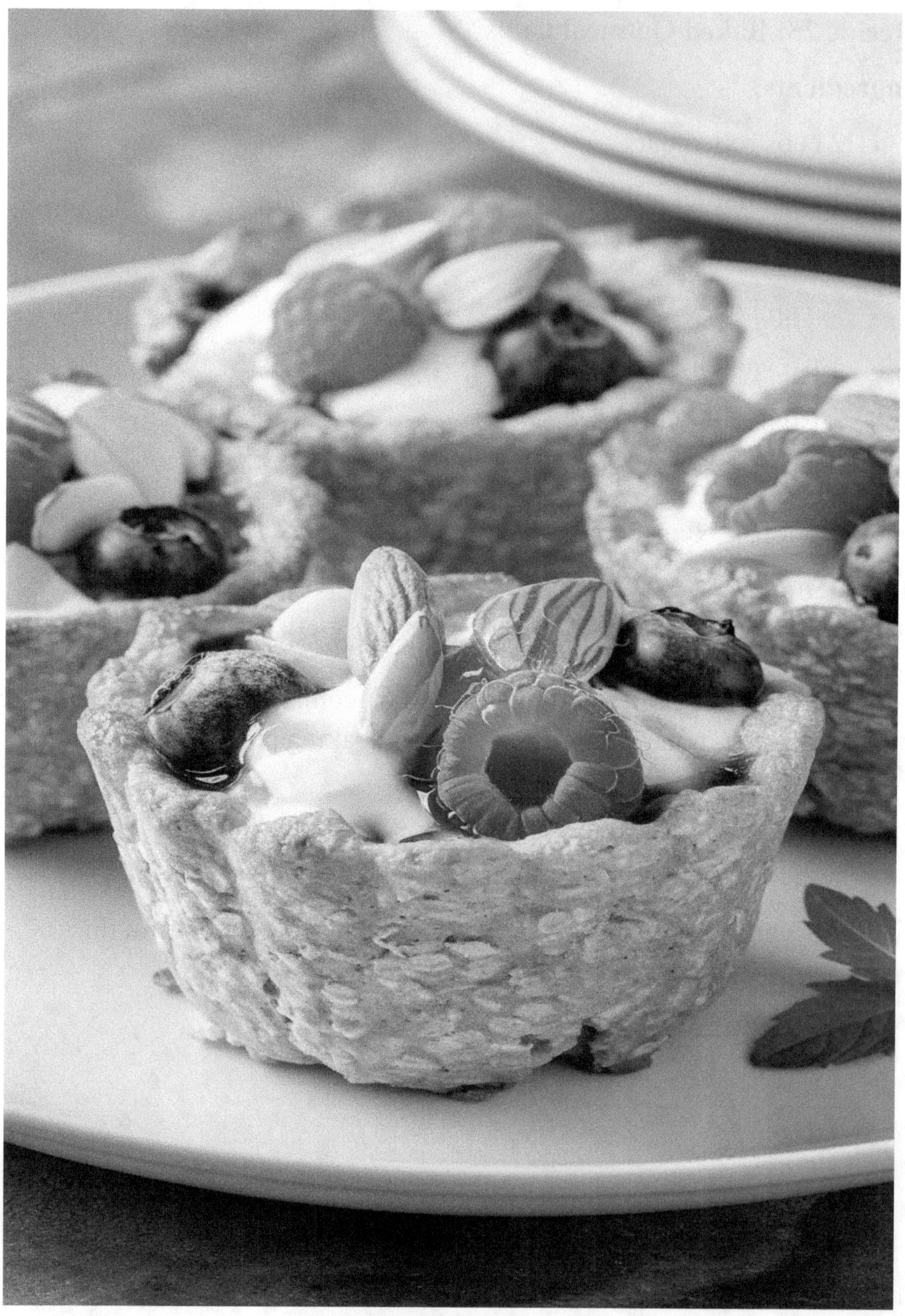